Writing for Publication in Nursing and Healthcare

Writing for Publication in Nursing and Healthcare

Getting It Right

Edited by

Karen Holland

Research Fellow
School of Nursing, Midwifery and Social Work
University of Salford
Salford
UK

Roger Watson

Professor of Nursing
Faculty of Health and Social Care
University of Hull
Hull
UK

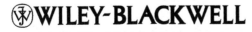

WILEY-BLACKWELL

A John Wiley & Sons, Ltd., Publication

Wiley-Blackwell is an imprint of John Wiley & Sons, formed by the merger of Wiley's global Scientific, Technical and Medical business with Blackwell Publishing.

Registered office: John Wiley & Sons, Ltd, The Atrium, Southern Gate, Chichester, West Sussex, PO19 8SQ, UK

Editorial offices: 9600 Garsington Road, Oxford, OX4 2DQ, UK
The Atrium, Southern Gate, Chichester, West Sussex, PO19 8SQ, UK
2121 State Avenue, Ames, Iowa 50014-8300, USA

For details of our global editorial offices, for customer services and for information about how to apply for permission to reuse the copyright material in this book please see our website at www.wiley.com/wiley-blackwell.

Library of Congress Cataloging-in-Publication Data
Writing for publication in nursing and healthcare : getting it right / edited by Karen Holland, Roger Watson.
      p. ; cm.
   Includes bibliographical references and index.
   ISBN 978-0-470-65782-9 (pbk. : alk. paper)
   I. Holland, Karen, 1949- II. Watson, Roger, 1955-
   [DNLM: 1. Writing-Nurses' Instruction.   2. Publishing-Nurses' Instruction. WZ 345]

   808.06′661-dc23
                                                                    2012011412

A catalogue record for this book is available from the British Library.

Wiley also publishes its books in a variety of electronic formats. Some content that appears in print may not be available in electronic books.

Cover images: main image - iStockphoto.com/© DNY59; patient/nurse image - iStockphoto.com/© deanm1974
Cover design by Meaden Creative

Set in 9/12.5 pt Interstate Light by Aptara® Inc., New Delhi, India

1   2012

Contents

List of Contributors

Editors

Karen Holland
Research Fellow
School of Nursing, Midwifery and Social Work
University of Salford
Salford
UK

Roger Watson
Professor of Nursing
Faculty of Health and Social Care
University of Hull
Hull
UK

Contributors

Seamus Cowman
Head of School of Nursing
Royal College of Surgeons in Ireland
Dublin
Ireland

Jan Draper
Head of Nursing
Department of Nursing
Faculty of Health and Social Care
The Open University
Milton Keynes
UK

Mark Hayter
Faculty of Health and Social Care
University of Hull
Hull
UK

Tracy Levett-Jones
Deputy Head of School (Teaching and Learning)
Lead – Research Centre for Health Professional Education
School of Nursing and Midwifery
Faculty of Health
University of Newcastle
Callaghan, NSW
Australia

Zena Moore
Lecturer in Wound Healing and Tissue Repair and Research Methodology
Programme Director
Faculty of Nursing and Midwifery
Royal College of Surgeons in Ireland
Dublin
Ireland

Paul Murphy
Royal College of Surgeons in Ireland
Dublin
Ireland

Charon A. Pierson
Editor-in-Chief, *Journal of the American Academy of Nurse Practitioners*
Director, Center for Aging
University of Texas
El Paso, TX
USA

Chantal F. Ski
Associate Professor
Cardiovascular Research Centre
Faculty of Health Sciences
Australian Catholic University
Melbourne, VIC
Australia

Teresa Stone
Senior Lecturer
School of Nursing and Midwifery
Faculty of Health
University of Newcastle
Callaghan, NSW
Australia

David R. Thompson
Professor of Nursing
Cardiovascular Research Centre
Faculty of Health Sciences
Australian Catholic University
Melbourne, VIC
Australia

Sue Turale
Editor-in-Chief, *Nursing and Health Sciences*
Fellow of the Royal College of Nursing Australia
Fellow of the Australian College of Mental Health Nurses
Professor of International Nursing
Yamaguchi University
Yamaguchi
Japan

Dean Whitehead
Senior Lecturer
School of Health and Social Services
Massey University
Palmerston North
Wellington
New Zealand

Foreword

It is a pleasure and privilege to be asked to write the foreword for this important book. It has arrived at an opportune time when there is a growing interest among health professionals in writing about their work and in understanding the mechanics of publishing.

Nurses and health professionals generally are members of applied disciplines, and the generation of knowledge is of little use if it is not disseminated. Our continued existence as a profession is based entirely on how we can improve the health and well-being of patients, their families and communities. The link between our knowledge base and our practice stands at the core of our survival as a discipline. As a result, we are extending our research and scholarly roles so as to provide evidence that underpins our practice and teaching. However, to produce such evidence without sharing it with others through publication and presentation is a fruitless exercise.

There are many reasons why health professionals publish. These include personal satisfaction, peer recognition or promotion of their career. Increasingly, health professionals in academia are expected to publish to promote scholarship or to have their research assessed. Currently, there are research assessment exercises in Australia, Finland, Hong Kong, New Zealand, Romania, Sweden and the United Kingdom. In each of these, the main element for consideration is publication. The old adage 'publish or perish' is more of a truism now than ever.

Publications take many forms, including everything from books, book chapters, book reviews, journal articles, editorials, conference papers, commentaries and letters. Both Karen Holland and Roger Watson have many years of experience in this field. Not only have they published extensively in all of the formats outlined above, they are also experienced editors and have boundless insight into the editorial process. They have assembled a number of high-profile contributors for this text from across the globe. Chapters cover everything from the basics of starting to write, to how publications are reviewed, to ethical and legal issues. I have always believed that the true experts in a subject are so comfortable with it that they can make it easily understandable. These contributors have this uncanny ability of simplifying the most complex of subjects. They do not have to dress the topic up in jargon and complicated terminology. They are also good storytellers and their stories of how ideas and research findings can be developed into publishable works will make readers come back to this text again and again.

The book is expertly crafted and its easy style and 'readability' are some of its most pleasing features. The activity boxes and key points give structure to the book as well as help engage its readers. Its slim volume will be acceptable to many health professionals who are turned off by some of the more heavier tomes on the subject. The short chapters are interesting and authoritative and can be read on a 'stand-alone' basis, allowing readers to 'dip in and out'.

So to my concluding remarks: I recommend with enthusiasm this text to would-be readers. It is a solid and significant contribution to the on-going development of our professions as generators and disseminators of knowledge.

Professor Hugh McKenna, CBE, PhD, BSc (Hons), RMN, RGN, RNT,
DipN(Lond), AdvDipEd, FFNRCSI, FEANS, FRCN, FAAN
Pro-Vice-Chancellor, Research and Innovation
University of Ulster

Preface

This book focuses on all aspects of writing for publication. It will help the reader to develop skills in writing articles, book reviews and other forms of publications but could also be viewed as an aide-memoire for editors and journal/book reviewers. 'Writing for publication' has become one of the most challenging phrases in nursing and midwifery language and practice, and is now seen as one of the essential prerequisites to a successful career in these professions. From personal experience of supporting colleagues to engage in the process of writing and to succeed in achieving their goal of a publication, we have developed various techniques and guidance that we use in workshops, study days and teaching and research activities.

As editors of two international nursing journals, we have also gained insight into and experience in the world of publishing, an experience that most of you reading this book will not have. This role has helped us to develop a range of skills to support individuals in writing for journals and attempting other forms of writing such as books, editorials or other forms of publication. By participating in these activities, it became clear that, despite the fact that there are textbooks that focus on certain aspects of writing for publication, there are few we could use that cover key aspects of both novice and expert needs. This book emerged from this need for a practical rather than theoretical approach to ensuring that, in using its content, individuals would be successful in writing for publication in different ways. This does not mean, however, that the book is without a strong evidence base, and there are many links to additional resources that can be accessed to support the writing and dissemination process. One of the fundamental aspects of any publication activity is also included: the ethical and legal aspects of publishing, which offers an invaluable guide to the pitfalls to avoid in developing good writing for publication practice.

The chapters are written by experts in the field: editors of journals, book authors and reviewers, article authors and reviewers, publishers and end-users of the academic and practice endeavours. They are also from the wider international scholarly community, bringing an added dimension of regional as well as international needs to be considered by the reader and user of the book.

The book offers the following unique aspects of knowledge and skills for successful publication:

(1) It covers the practical 'how to do it' with the theoretical principles and rules that govern academic writing, publishing and dissemination.

(2) It can be used by readers worldwide not only in the disciplines of nursing and midwifery but also in other healthcare professions.

(3) It uses examples to illustrate the practical ways in which abstracts, papers, book reviews and other sorts of publications can be written and disseminated.

(4) Helpful tips on what to do and what not to do are also included.

(5) It offers key principles of writing for publication, which can be adapted to different scenarios and opportunities.

There are 16 chapters, each written by colleagues who have achieved varying degrees of success in writing for publication and most importantly the dissemination of knowledge, which has an impact on the various fields of clinical practice as well as education, management and further research. The chapters cover most types of writing for publication activities, and the content can be adapted to suit other forms of writing for publication not covered in depth in this book. A bibliography is offered at the end of the book for more specific reading and guidance.

Chapter 1 offers an explanation of why these chapters are included and our philosophy in writing the book itself, the title of which (*Writing for Publication in Nursing and Healthcare: Getting It Right*) illustrates what we hope will be an invaluable resource for both new and experienced authors in their quest for successful publication activity.

Karen Holland, Editor of *Nurse Education in Practice*
Roger Watson, Editor-in-Chief of *Journal of Advanced Nursing*
January 2012

Acknowledgements

Our own journey in *Writing for Publication in Nursing and Healthcare* has been one of many challenges in our professional careers, but we have both been fortunate to encounter mentors and support along the way. It is opportune, therefore, that this book especially enables us to thank particular individuals who have been instrumental in promoting the field of nursing and midwifery scholarship internationally.

Roger would like to thank Dr James P. Smith OBE, founding Editor of *Journal of Advanced Nursing*, for the opportunity to become involved with academic publishing and his early and continuing guidance on his career and progress. He would also like to thank Wiley-Blackwell for their continued tolerance and indulgence in his career as an editor.

Karen would like to acknowledge, with grateful thanks, the support given by Professor Peter Birchenall in giving her the opportunity 12 years ago to learn alongside him how to become an editor. His support and guidance enabled her to have the confidence to promote the development of *Nurse Education in Practice* (an Elsevier journal) and become its first editor.

We would both like to thank all our chapter contributors who have also been on their own 'writing journeys', and also make a significant contribution to the promotion of good practice in various forms of publications and scholarship. We are grateful that they have been able to find the time to share their knowledge and experience with us and you, the reader of this book.

Finally, we wish to acknowledge Magenta Styles from Wiley-Blackwell who has given us this opportunity to be self-indulgent and edit a book on a topic close to our interests and enjoyment, and to the whole of the publication team, especially Sarah Claridge (Editorial Assistant) for her patience and support, Nick and Amit for their support with the 'finishing touches' of editing and proof reading processes, and also Liz Lyons for the fabulous book cover design.

Karen Holland, Editor of *Nurse Education in Practice*
Roger Watson, Editor-in-Chief of *Journal of Advanced Nursing*

Chapter 1

Introduction: The Book, Its Philosophy and Its Focus

Karen Holland[1] and Roger Watson[2]

[1]School of Nursing, Midwifery and Social Work, University of Salford, Salford, UK
[2]Faculty of Health and Social Care, University of Hull, Hull, UK

Introduction

The use of evidence has become a central part of both faculty (academia) and professional practice. For many, it has become a core element of their career development and opportunity for advancement. Therefore, producing this evidence has become an essential skill for nursing and midwifery academics and qualified practitioners; one that all undergraduate and postgraduate students need to develop as part of their curriculum and for their future careers.

Disseminating the evidence once it has been produced is at the core of this book, and we will not enter into philosophical debates on the nature of what is best evidence and what we do to obtain the evidence itself, nor about which approach is best for dissemination. This book is, arguably, a body of evidence in its own right; one that has collected a range of views and supporting material on writing for publication, different approaches and – most importantly – how to help you translate your ideas, opinions and research findings into meaningful dialogue with those who will want to read them and hopefully influence and contribute to the development of their professional practice.

This written evidence is found in a range of published works: books, peer-reviewed articles, opinion papers and research reports. Therefore, 'getting this right' with regard to writing for publication becomes essential for the future scholarship of the nursing and midwifery professions as well as the evidence-based rigour underpinning professional practice.

However, in the twenty-first century the 'written' word is no longer the main form of communication; technological advances enable us to disseminate research evidence and other forms of scholarly endeavour in numerous

Writing for Publication in Nursing and Healthcare: Getting It Right, First Edition.
Edited by Karen Holland and Roger Watson.
© 2012 John Wiley & Sons, Ltd. Published 2012 by John Wiley & Sons, Ltd.

innovative ways, but which has also brought with it many new challenges. Maybe, we should now consider 'desktop typing for publication' as an adjunct to 'writing for publication', and offer the basics on not only how to write but also how to use the technology to engage in the dissemination of scholarship. Watson in Chapter 2 of this book refers to some of the practical issues of using a computer in the writing process.

Why publish what we write?

Although publishing in various forms is about sharing best practice and evidence of various kinds, we publish for other reasons. Many of you reading this will recall situations where you read something in a newspaper article that you disagreed with or something you feel strongly about and wished you had the courage to write a letter to the newspaper in reply (see Chapter 16). You may even have reached the stage of having written the letter, but something held you back and you did not send it; possibly having second thoughts that, maybe, the language was too strong!

In many journals, there are opportunities for a similar kind of communications, especially as editorials or guest editorials where, again, it is about having a strong or opposing view on a topic that you feel needs to be raised, resulting often in being a trigger for other responses to be published to further debate (if the editor allows!) or in some cases ideas for further research.

Many clinical practitioners will be developing new ways of nursing that others could benefit from, and unlike in the past, where publishing anything was viewed as the province of 'academia' or faculty staff, there has been a major shift in who is writing for publication. Publishing what you write is no longer the province of the few, evident by the plethora of journals published worldwide.

For colleagues in many countries, having the opportunity to publish what they write is not easy; in particular, where English is not the first language, they may not have journals to write in and most importantly no large publishers to take on the risk of developing new journals or publishing new books in an area such as nursing, which is still developing in many countries. This development also involves the undertaking of research, the writing and dissemination of their work in their own country and, most importantly, sharing this with the international community in their own discipline.

One country that is taking the risk, and publishing a new nursing journal, is Lithuania, with colleagues at the Lithuanian University of Health Sciences in Kaunas publishing their first issue of the journal *Nursing Education, Research and Practice* in September of 2011. The editorial by the editor-in-chief and the dean of the Faculty of Nursing highlights a very important reason for why they are supporting the promotion of publishing what their colleagues write, in relation to where they are in the 'bigger picture' of what most of us have taken for granted:

> [T]he journal specifically aims to become a platform available for East-
> ern European countries with post-Soviet nursing and midwifery systems to
> share new ideas and demonstrate rapid and significant advancements in the
> nursing and midwifery disciplines.
>
> (Macijauskiene and Stankevicius, 2011, p. 1)

Given the fact that the journal was also published at a time of celebrating the 20th anniversary of their Faculty of Nursing, they should be congratulated on this achievement alone, let alone beginning a new journey in publishing what their peers have been writing about in isolation from each other. For many countries and disciplines worldwide, the question 'why publish what we write?' is more than simply a question of having to publish, but retains some of the altruistic stance that many of us began with in relation to helping others through sharing our knowledge and evidence as well-perceived wisdom.

For others, publishing what we write becomes an employment necessity with many jobs requiring applicants to have undertaken research and also published papers in journals. For others, retaining their posts also requires the same criteria, and this is often even more challenging for colleagues and takes them very often outside their 'comfort zone' both in terms of confidence in their abilities to write anything for publication and also needing additional skills to be gained to maximise their chances for success. Others among you will be postgraduate or even undergraduate students, for whom writing elements of their theses or dissertations becomes an integral part of that studentship. Many of you will be expected to write with your supervisors as a continuous process, but most of you will have a publication plan built into your personal and professional learning plans, including publishing at least one or two of your papers in a peer-reviewed international journal. For many undergraduate students, having an opportunity to write for publication may take a different form, as seen in the *Nursing Standard* journal (Lee, 2011, p. 29) where students write their reflection and actions as a result of a practice experience in the 'the real world of nursing'. This is an excellent starting point for the future in managing time, writing and also helping others to learn through their experiences.

We hope that this book will enable this group to gain in confidence and skills, while the more experienced colleagues will use it more for 'branching out' into new areas of publishing their work. Seeing your work, whatever form it takes, in print or electronically for the first time or in a different medium is a wonderful feeling and, in fact, for many of us that initial 'buzz' never really goes away. Mainly, it is because we remain committed, especially as editors, to writing and sharing our knowledge and experience with others, as well as actually enjoying the writing itself. It is not quite the same as having to write to order, when it possibly can be seen as a chore!

Therefore, if publishing what we write is important, either politically or professionally, why do so many people still find it hard to achieve success or even get off the ground?

What are perceived barriers to successful writing?

In the chapters in this book, you will find examples of why individuals either set up barriers themselves to writing for publication or find obstacles placed in front of them. Many reasons also overlap and are often a combination of both. As mentioned, many of us have to begin somewhere, and all of us writing in this book will have come across barriers of one kind and another since we began to see our work being published for others to read and the material being used in some way in their work or their professional development.

To say that writing for publication is easy would not be the whole truth; however, depending on what you are writing and who you are writing for, some people find some forms of writing much easier than others. This could be writing an article for some, writing a book for others or writing conference abstracts and papers. Some of you reading this in order to learn new skills or knowledge may well be saying, 'it's all right for them, as they already do it', but even for us there are always new things to learn, and in today's publishing climate, there are new media to try out in terms of publishing what we write about.

Barriers written about in other books on writing for publication or articles in journals include:

- time and effort to write;
- difficulty in writing down what you need to say;
- lack of skills in writing for different audiences;
- lack of awareness of what is required for successful publication;
- 'writer's block' – situations where not only it is difficult to write anything at all but also you may be under pressure to write to a deadline and 'your mind goes blank' and panic sets in.

And one that most of us fear when first starting on this 'writing journey', and that is:

- fear of rejection – of having your work rejected and, therefore, self-perception that you have been rejected as well as the actual publication.

With all these barriers that could be affecting your personal commitment to write for publication, how can you be successful in your writing endeavours? Overcoming these barriers is considered in Chapter 2.

How can we succeed?

Books like this one will give you a basic foundation in learning 'how to be successful' at writing for publication. We will offer you links to numerous resources that will support a successful outcome of seeing your work published in a variety of different media, but all of which rely on the message you wish to convey and who the audience or readership is.

However, successful publication will for most of you take time to develop but for others it will be as with all those drivers who pass their test the first time, simply putting pen to paper (some of us still do use pen/pencil and paper to write down initial thoughts and outlines!) and writing 'just happens'! These are probably the rare ones but having known some of these they also can 'get stuck', and here they may enlist the help of colleagues.

Successful publishing will depend on some kind of review process, even in writing books or book chapters, and this is a positive aspect of the writing process. Asking a colleague with publishing experience or even asking someone who would be reading your work in a journal is an essential part of developing skills and expertise as an author in whatever capacity. Receiving critique from a colleague on your writing also enables you to refine and revise your paper/book chapter, if necessary, to ensure that, when an article, for example, is published, there is an increased likelihood of it achieving publication.

In addition to achieving success with an actual publication, it is important to consider that there are other things you can do in terms of developing successful writing skills as well as strategies when you are actually writing. Most of these are considered in the following chapters, and certain skills will apply to some and not others. One of the fundamental issues that crosses all of them is the good time management, including setting time aside specifically for writing on your own or writing with others.

Different media for publication will, of course, also have an impact on your writing for publication – and the use of various forms of technology and images as 'writing' is becoming more evident. Technology is to be found in articles themselves as well, through linking to other publications in reference lists as direct access links, and even technology within papers online to illustrate meaning and purpose.

Technology is now the main medium for actual submission of articles themselves, and book manuscripts are no longer sent ring bound to publishers in multiple copies and floppy discs. Regardless of how to convey the messages of our publications, the key is what the message is initially and this will tell us how and what we write as well as where and to whom we send the messages.

Summary

This book can be viewed as a 'lens' into these different kinds of writing media, as well as helping you understand and work with the processes involved in each case. It is also about giving you the confidence either to try something new or to try writing in any form for the first time.

We have experienced co-authors writing from their personal experiences for you. None is an expert at everything, but between us all we have a collective experience and enjoyment of both writing for publication itself and sharing that with you. The title of the book is *Writing for Publication in Nursing and*

Healthcare: Getting It Right – we like to think that we can both help you on this journey and also travel with you on the journey. As editors ourselves, we are very much aware of how hard getting it right and being successful at writing itself are, and we look forward to feedback from you following publication.

References

Lee, S. (2011) Boundaries between nurses and patients must be clearly defined, student experiences in the real world of nursing. *Nursing Standard*, 26(4), 29.

Macijauskiene, J. & Stankevicius, E. (2011) *Editorial, Nursing Education, Research & Practice*. Kaunas: Lithuanian University of Health Sciences.

Further reading

Gimenez, J. (2011) *Writing for Nursing and Midwifery Students*, 2nd edition. Basingstoke: Palgrave Macmillan.
Although aimed at an undergraduate readership, it is a useful book for those endeavouring to write for publication for the first time and also for potential authors where English is not the first language. It explains how to write in a number of different kinds of formats (genres) and offers clarity in terms of glossary of terms used in both academic writing and publishing articles.

Webb, C. (2009) Writing for Publication: an easy to follow guide for any nurse thinking of publishing their work, Nurse Author Editor journal. Available at: http://www.nurseauthoreditor.com/WritingforPublication2009.pdf [Accessed 12 April 2012].

Websites

The Nurse Author Editor website for authors, editors and reviewers and edited by one of our chapter editors, Dr Charon A. Pierson. Available at: http://www.nurseauthoreditor.com/ [Accessed 7 October 2011].

These are links to Elsevier publication websites information for authors. Available at: http://www.elsevier.com/wps/find/authorsview.authors/landing_main [Accessed 12 April 2012] and http://www.nursingplus.com/ [Accessed 12 April 2012] (also has additional resource links to Nurse Author Editor material).

Chapter 2

The Basics of Writing for Publication and the Steps to Success: Getting Started

Roger Watson

Faculty of Health and Social Care, University of Hull, Hull, UK

Introduction

This chapter covers some of the essential features of writing an article for publication, taking into account the barriers that some people feel about writing and how to overcome these. While the chapter focuses on writing an original article, many of the principles apply to other forms of writing, for example book chapters and reviews, and these will be covered in the subsequent chapters.

Barriers to writing

I teach an online unit of study on information and communication in healthcare with several sessions on writing for publication. One of the first exercises I set for the students - mostly busy clinicians who want to write - is to list their perceived barriers to writing and to share this with the group online, and with me. The list grows longer every time I do this exercise as people find endless reasons not to write, despite their desire to do so. However, in every list and somewhere near the top in terms of 'popularity' are the following:

- Lack of time
- Lack of ability
- Not understanding the publishing process
- Fear of criticism
- Fear of rejection

Writing for Publication in Nursing and Healthcare: Getting It Right, First Edition.
Edited by Karen Holland and Roger Watson.
© 2012 John Wiley & Sons, Ltd. Published 2012 by John Wiley & Sons, Ltd.

Lack of time

This is always the top reason people perceive as the main barrier to writing. Naturally, writing takes time and time becomes scarcer as we progress through our working lives. The myriad advances that could help us to write – primarily the word-processing facilities of personal computers – instead provide us with myriad distractions: email, the World Wide Web, Facebook and Twitter. We rarely have the time we think that it takes to write a substantial piece of work (but more about time later), and one thing is certain, that is, nobody is going to give us the time. Therefore, when we are in a position to have something to write about, for example through experience and seniority, we often lack the time to do it. However, some people write frequently and copiously and they do not seem to have appreciably more time on their hands than anyone else. We may well ask – how do they do it? Of course, there is no one simple answer to this question as we will see throughout this book.

Lack of ability

This is a major fear that is seen as a barrier to writing. This fear stems from lack of experience and opportunity and also, sadly, from bad experiences of having your early efforts at writing dismissed by teachers, lecturers, friends and colleagues. People who have this fear will have done the minimum necessary to 'get through' their education at school, college or university and will have gladly left writing behind, until they are in a situation where some writing is required or they re-develop a desire to write. I hope that, in these pages, anyone with such a fear will find the means to overcome it and also to withstand the inevitable and necessary critical review of their work that is an essential part of writing. Clearly, lack of experience is a barrier to writing, but everyone who writes regularly lacked experience at some point (Salwak, 2011) and it is towards this end that this chapter, and indeed the whole book, is written. In this chapter, I hope to share how I do it. However, not everything I say will apply to you and not everything may work for you either, but based on the principles expressed, it would be good to know that you have made an attempt.

Not understanding the publishing process

Like all unfamiliar processes, the publishing process has some of its own procedures and terminology (jargon if you like). To have something published properly, you need to have a publisher, and this brings you into contact with a wide range of people and roles you will never have encountered: editors, editors-in-chief and production editors, for example, to be considered in Chapter 11. You will encounter entities such as manuscripts, proofs, copyright agreements and a relatively new development such as digital object identifiers. Publishing is an industry and, while publishers are interested in helping people to publish and do take a genuine interest in this work, publishing companies must make a profit, and the whole process from submission to production is tightly controlled and replicated across different publishing companies.

Learning about the publishing process

I am not recommending that you make a deliberate effort to learn about the publishing industry and the people working in it; mostly your contact will be with an editor and you will mainly be concerned with your manuscript and the proof (the article version that looks like the final product but still requires correction). You will learn about other aspects of publishing as you become more experienced at writing for publication, and the objective of this chapter is to help you to gain a general insight only.

Writing for publication in what are known as 'scientific' journals is mainly a technical process. On the whole, it is not the same as creative writing, such as writing a magazine story, although good technical writing and good creative writing share many of the same features. Mainly, you will know what you want to write about, for example the outcome of a research study, an opinion about something that interests or has irritated you or something that you have been asked to write because you are a recognised expert.

Experience only comes from doing something (King, 2004) and doing something only happens when you make a start. Therefore, in the face of the common barriers to writing mentioned above, the aim of this chapter is to help you to make a start and overcome these barriers.

Getting started

Getting started essentially depends on your motivation to write and these motivations include self-motivation, obligation to write (e.g. as an academic seeking promotion) or the imposition of a deadline. It is impossible to say which is the best motivation factor because everyone is different and everyone responds differently to these motivations. However, whatever the source, there is often a period of adjustment to the task of writing and this often involves staring at a blank computer screen or for some of us just looking blank!

When you have made a start to writing you have, by virtue of doing it, overcome the main barrier: lack of time. But how did you do it? Clearly, you must have set aside some time or possibly 'borrowed' or 'stolen' time from some other activity. But how much time and how much progress did you make?

A common mistake, in my experience, is to set aside whole days, weeks or even months for writing. Very few people can sustain writing for more than an hour or so at a time, even full-time authors rarely write all day. Therefore, time set aside in a large amount for writing is often wasted time – writing is hard work but you do not need a rest after doing it; what you need is a change and it is more sensible to fit small, regular and frequent times for writing into your normal working day. You may feel that you do not have any time in your normal working day; however, do you really work every minute of every hour you are at work? How about the half hour before everyone else arrives and the telephone starts ringing? How about the last half hour of the day or just remaining for an extra half hour to do some writing? The same goes for being at home – we all have busy personal lives but there are free periods before going to work, after arriving home from work or before going to bed. I am not suggesting all of these options or any of these in particular; they are merely some suggestions. At first, you may seem to be making little progress, but this is where the 'four rules' of writing apply. These will be 'unpacked' for you in order to guide the 'getting started' process.

The 'four rules' of writing

The four rules of writing as expressed here are mine (Watson, 2011), although I do not claim to be the first to think of them, nor do I claim copyright. Many writers will express how they write in a series of hints or rules and many will say the same thing: a cursory search on Google for 'the four rules of writing' will yield a series of 'hits'. I only take credit for bringing together these particular four points and labelling them as such. I describe these as 'rules' without wishing to appear dogmatic; these are not all that you need to do to write but I call them 'rules' because I simply cannot see how, by applying these as a minimum set of guidelines, you can fail to produce some writing.

Please note that these are not rules for writing well – but without doing some writing, you cannot write well; these rules – especially the first two – will help you to fill a few pages and make a start to getting them into 'shape'. Once you have written something, you can work to improve it, and we will look at how that is done later. The 'four rules' of writing are shown in Box 2.1.

Rule 1: Read the guidelines

The author guidelines for journals are easily available on the publisher website on the Internet and you must consult these with regard to the permitted length of the article, the general layout and other conventions that need to be followed (Miser, 1998). Some examples of guidelines to popular nursing journals are provided in Box 2.2. Specific aspects of the guidelines will be examined in Chapter 5.

Rule 2: Set targets and count words

Without exception, when I have asked other good writers about writing or listened to another writer giving a presentation on writing, they have referred

---

Box 2.1 The four rules of writing

(1) Read the guidelines (see Chapter 5).
(2) Set targets and count words.
(3) Seek criticism.
(4) Treat rejection as the beginning of the next submission.

> **Box 2.2**   Link to journal guidelines (accessed 10 July 2011)
>
> *International Journal of Nursing Studies*: http://www.elsevier.com/wps/ find/journaldescription.cws_home/266/authorinstructions
> *Journal of Advanced Nursing*: http://onlinelibrary.wiley.com/journal/ 10.1111/(ISSN)1365-2648/homepage/ForAuthors.html
> *Journal of Clinical Nursing*: http://onlinelibrary.wiley.com/journal/ 10.1111/(ISSN)1365-2702/homepage/ForAuthors.html
> *Nurse Education in Practice*: http://www.elsevier.com/wps/find/journal description.cws_home/623062/authorinstructions
> *Nurse Education Today*: http://www.elsevier.com/wps/find/journalde scription.cws_home/623061/authorinstructions

to setting targets as an essential step. Some professional writers, such as popular novelists, have enormous targets – in the thousands of words – but these are very experienced writers who do it full-time and depend on their writing to earn a living. They can write quickly and will have meticulously researched their topic and immersed themselves almost exclusively in it. Most of us are not 'immersed' in our writing in the same way; while we may be preoccupied with it, we have other things such as clinical work, teaching, research and meetings to fit into our working day. Therefore, applying the idea suggested above about 'snatching' short periods of time to write, we should set commensurately sensible and achievable targets.

Targets are personal and my suggestion is that you make them reasonable so that you achieve some writing but not too large an amount or you will not meet them. My personal target is 500 words every time I sit down to write; sometimes that is every day over a prolonged period but, with regular interruptions and long periods when writing is difficult, it is essential to have a target each time you find time to write. Of course, this will depend on what kind of publication you are writing and word length required. Many chapters in this book will help you to focus on word limits and various forms of dissemination activities.

When you reach your target... stop!

This is also something that many writers say, and the idea is that your targets must be real, as well as being realistic: there is no need to go beyond them when you achieve them (Hodson, 2007). The danger, even when you are doing well with a piece of writing, is that you will try to progress beyond your target and fail to achieve it; this way you will end up being disappointed. Sometimes, you think you can continue but you either run out of ideas or you find it hard to express them; in this case, it is essential to stop and do something else.

For example, when I was writing this chapter, I reached the end of the section before the sub-heading above and felt that I could continue. The section ended neatly at 1500 words, representing three writing sessions. In fact, I was unable

Box 2.3 Writing down bullet points

- Reach target and stop.
- Count the words.
- How to fill a blank page.

to continue as I was tired and did not have the time; therefore, I applied another useful technique. I wrote a few bullet points with ideas for the section you are currently reading at the end of the section I had just written (Box 2.3). However, you can also use a notebook for this and you will find one a very useful thing to carry with you if you are serious about writing. I find this works well as it ensures that you have not lost your ideas, and you have made some progress with the next section. Most importantly, it gives you a 'thread' to pick up when you return to the piece of writing; all you have to do is 'flesh out' or expand the bullet point headings and sometimes this gives you your next 500 words and the process continues.

Count words

I constantly count the number of words I am writing and, of course, this is easy with the word counting facility in word-processing packages. Counting words is important for two reasons: all writing is undertaken to a prescribed number of words (commonly 5000 words for an original article); therefore, you need to know how you are progressing. Counting words is also encouraging; every time you write another sentence you have increased the word count and you can follow progress easily. As the number of words grows, counting the words positively reinforces your endeavours; counting the words also tells you when to stop.

Of course, sometimes your ideas do not flow onto the screen; we all get stuck and there is a temptation to stop short of our target. Do not give in to this temptation. My advice is to think ahead as explained in the next section. For your information, I reached 2005 words at the end of the last sentence and was also running out of ideas so - again - I am leaving in the bullet points I wrote down for your information in Boxes 2.3 and 2.4, and you will see how I used these in the next section. Before reading on, you might want to try the exercise in Box 2.5.

Box 2.4 More bullet points

- Do not get stuck - do the next section.
- Write the headings in first.
- Do not worry too much what you are writing.
- *Never* write on paper, only on screen.

Box 2.5 Write 500 words now

Choose a topic that you know something about; for example, from your own clinical practice or teaching and, without stopping, write 500 words about it.

How to fill a blank page

The writer's enemy is the blank page – or the blank screen in the case of the personal computer. The secret to filling pages is not to worry too much what you are writing at the time. Remember, you can edit a bad page of writing but you cannot edit a blank page. Therefore, whatever relevant ideas to the topic you are addressing are in your head, get them typed as soon as you can. Sometimes we get stuck, and we do not know what to write next. My advice here is to move to the next section or, if the writing is advanced, then move back a section and see if anything needs to be added to increase the word count.

It is very helpful, and this especially applies to writing articles, if you type in all the headings that you will use in the manuscript and give these a page each and separate them by a page break, and type them in bold and capital letters to find them easily. A typical set of headings is shown in Box 2.6. However, you should note that journals differ slightly in the headings that they require, and therefore, it is essential that you check the specific guidelines for the journal you are writing for. Before proceeding, you may want to try the exercise in Box 2.7.

Box 2.6 Typical headings for a manuscript

Title
Abstract
Introduction
Background
Methods
Results
Discussion

Box 2.7 Exercise: create a file and headings

Why not create a word-processing file now and save it with an appropriate label, for example 'Latest Publication', and then insert a set of headings, as suggested in the text, and then you will have started your first manuscript.

Many journals prescribe the headings so you do not have to think about this, and remember that, it is not necessary or advisable to start at the beginning and work your way through the manuscript in that order. For example, you may have a few ideas for the abstract that you can type in, but it is better to leave the abstract until the end – then you know what you are abstracting. The abstract may also have sub-headings that the journal will give you; if not, then it is a good idea to use sub-headings for the abstract – they can always be removed prior to submission (Watson, 2006). Often, this skeleton of what your article is going to be, with a provisional title to guide you, is enough for one writing session. Rather than trying to fill the blanks immediately, it may be wise to leave this for the next session and then you can begin in earnest. I will return to what should appear under each of these headings in Chapter 5.

Once you have started, when you get stuck, as you certainly will at some point, just jump to another section and write something relevant there. Remember to count the words and you will see that you are making progress and, of course, stop when you reach your target. In relation to making progress with writing it is essential that you learn, if you have not already adopted the habit, of writing directly into a word-processing package.

Some 'old timers', or those who have not been converted to technology, who are established authors will disagree, and it took me some time to be convinced about this. But just look at the benefits: this is a single keystroke process, and you do not have to find time to copy type your work into a computer (type in from the copy of the written material). Related to the last point, you may never make or find that time and, if you have tried it, copy typing is very hard work (I still have not completed the transcription of the diary I kept while serving in the First Gulf War – that was in 1990!). You can count the words and begin to edit on screen and you have a permanent copy; but do not be naïve about this, do make backup copies of all your work. This can be through copying your work directly onto a separate hard drive linked to your computer, or onto a USB data stick. Make sure that all your files are labelled correctly in your filing system, and that each time you save something that the actual version is numbered and copied! Many of us have on occasion struggled to find the right version of something we have written because of inattention to this, causing some stress when you imagine you have lost all that you have written the day before, only to find you have labelled it as something else instead. Getting started for writing involves more than just 'thinking' preparation; it also involves a different way of working with regard to writing or in relation to the computer word processing.

I am not saying that you should never write anything down on a manuscript or a piece of paper; on the contrary, I find a small notebook or journal that can slip easily into a travel bag or brief case very useful for noting down ideas as they come to me on trains and planes, when my portable computer is not available.

And a final tip, if you can afford it, is to invest in a portable computer (or an electronic notebook) that really is portable – small and light – that can be easily carried in hand luggage. As you become busier, and as you write more, you will rarely have the luxury of sitting at your desk at home or in the office to write. It is good practice not to develop a favourite place to write – learn to write wherever you are, especially while travelling. It fills the time and fills pages.

Rule 3: Seek critical review

Once you have written your first draft, it is time to begin editing your work. Even the most experienced writers rarely get it right first time: some revision and editing of your work is essential (Salwak, 2011). The main point of the process described above is to have something to edit. However, be assured that the more you write, the better you will become at getting it right in fewer drafts.

There is no limit to what you can do with your own editing. You will have to check simple things like spelling; do not trust the word-processing spellchecker or grammar checker entirely (words like 'net' and 'ten' are easily mistyped for each other and not recognised as mistake). On the other hand, do investigate any apparent anomalies that the word-processing package indicates; many people do not.

Otherwise, check the grammar and the expression of phrases and sentences to make sure they make sense; try to remove unnecessary words (see Chapter 5) and generally make sure that the work is organised logically. This editing process may take several sessions. Once you have edited a complete draft, do not return to the beginning and start again at the same sitting; it really pays to set the work aside for a while and return to it later. Once you are happy with your own writing and editing you are ready for the next essential step, which is to show it to someone else. It is excellent practice to seek critical review of your work, and even the most experienced writers do this. As an editor, it is easy to see who has not taken this advice prior to submission of an article. In Chapter 5 you will see an example where if the authors had done so, they may well have improved their chances of success.

About seeking critical review

It is never easy seeking criticism, or an opinion, and it always carries some risks; we all need help with writing and most of us want it, but we do not like to ask. We are afraid of adverse comments, but if you bear the following points in mind, then it should make it easier for you, and like writing itself, the more you seek criticism, the easier you will accept it, while becoming a better writer and requiring fewer adverse comments and changes.

A good point to remember is that, if you are writing for publication (whether it is an article or a book chapter), you are not writing for yourself; you are writing for other people. For this reason, other people are the best judges of your writing. Therefore, once you are happy with your first draft, find someone to read it; better still, find more than one person. The optimum number in my view is two people; it can be helpful to get more than one perspective but it helps not to be 'bombarded' with too many comments.

I find that experienced writing colleagues and less experienced writing colleagues are equally helpful, but for different reasons. Experienced colleagues will often have submitted to the same journal as you are targeting and will have comments about the overall structure and the quality of the arguments; they may also know what some editors and journals like. Less experienced colleagues, and sometimes people unrelated to the topic you are writing about, will often ask, repeatedly, 'what does that mean?' or point out 'this doesn't make sense', and will often spot minor errors that you have overlooked. This is all valuable criticism.

You must learn to accept the criticism and not take it personally; the criticism should be about your writing and not about you. Even negative comments are, ultimately, positive if they help you to have your work published. Bear in mind that, if you do not get suitable criticism at this stage, you will get it from reviewers of your work and from editors, with potentially more serious outcomes, often with a rejection of your manuscript. While nothing guarantees acceptance, you should be aware that the most common reason for rejection is poor writing, and you want to get over that hurdle if you can and have your manuscript read for its substance and not rejected for its presentation (Sullivan, 2002). Likewise, if you are asked to criticise someone's writing, you must be willing to do it; this is something you will get better and quicker at as you gain more experience. You may at the end of the experience have enough confidence to become a reviewer for a journal (see Chapter 12).

Whom to ask for critical review

Do ask people whom you trust: you need to be sure that you are going to get criticism of your writing and not you; do not ask people who are always negative - it is absolutely no use if you know that someone always gives negative feedback and is also destructive and not constructive. However, do not seek criticism from someone who is afraid to give it either. At the other end of the spectrum, the kind of person who hands you back your work with no suggested changes and always compliments you on it is not very helpful. Your writing is rarely perfect, and there is always room for improvement; even for the most experienced of writers. Very rarely will authors be able to have an article accepted without any changes (see Chapter 5).

Rule 4: Treat rejection as the beginning of the next submission

The fourth rule of writing is an essential part of the process - especially for academic journals: treat rejection as the beginning of the next submission. If your manuscript is rejected by one journal, then there is nothing to prevent you from submitting it elsewhere. It is nearly universal to assign copyright to the publisher to whom you submit a manuscript at the point of submission, but if the manuscript is rejected, then the copyright is re-assigned to you and you must not give up. (Keeping rejected articles in a drawer without doing anything with them is not helpful, neither to yourself nor indeed to the reviewers who may have taken time to give constructive feedback.) It helps, nevertheless, to understand the reasons for rejection, in order to be able to consider the next steps (see Chapter 5).

Reasons for rejection

The most common reasons for rejection of manuscripts is poor writing (Sullivan, 2002), and it is possible that your manuscript has been rejected for this reason. If you observe the third rule of writing (seeking criticism), you should minimise this reason for rejection, but there are no guarantees. However, if you assume that your manuscript is well written, then there are many reasons for rejection, and these will be considered in more detail in Chapter 5.

However, it is important to appreciate that journals are usually under a great deal of pressure for space in terms of the number of articles they are able to publish in any one issue or volume (i.e. number of issues in any given year).

Less-established journals that receive few manuscripts tend to be quite small and, in addition, often have less space to publish articles. They may also become less popular as a result. On the other hand, well-established journals that are very popular, while they are bigger and are published more frequently, often receive manuscripts far in excess of the space available (see Chapter 5). For example, when I was an editor with *Journal of Clinical Nursing* we received approximately three times as many manuscripts in a year than we could publish; for journals like the *BMJ* (*British Medical Journal*), it is approximately ten times. When this happens, if a journal continues to accept the majority of these manuscripts, then authors are kept waiting for long periods, sometimes years, before their article is published (in paper-based format) and the information in it is out of date when it is published. However, the introduction of electronic submission of articles means that, immediately the article proofs are corrected, the article can be published in an electronic format on the journal website prior to being published in the paper-based version. Examples of these are Articles in Press (*Nurse Education in Practice* - Elsevier: http://www.sciencedirect.com/science/journal/aip/14715953) and Early View (*Journal of Advanced Nursing* - Wiley-Blackwell: http://online library.wiley.com/journal/10.1111/(ISSN)1365-2648/earlyview).

Therefore, to accommodate the large numbers of manuscripts submitted, the only action a journal editor can take is to reject more manuscripts to speed up publication and make the contents more current. This should also increase the quality of the articles in the journal as the editor can then select the manuscripts that are more relevant to the journal and are of the highest quality. Therefore, your manuscript may be rejected because it does not impress the editor on submission or, if it is sent out for review, any criticism from the reviewers is likely to result in rejection (see Chapters 11 and 12). If the manuscript has been sent out for review, then it is likely to be returned with some feedback giving the reasons for rejection; you should consider and incorporate this feedback when possible in the process of submitting elsewhere.

The process of submitting, reviewing and rejecting or accepting manuscripts for publication is not a scientific process (Russell, 2010); at each stage,

individuals are involved and these are all being asked to exercise their professional and personal judgement. Therefore, there is no guaranteed way of
achieving publication and predicting the comments that you may receive.
However, as you will see in Chapters 11 and 12, the editor of any journal has significant decision-making to do when determining the nature of the feedback
to authors. Destructive feedback is not helpful to either new or established
authors and their role is to ensure that authors do not stop writing before
really getting started.

The process of publishing

To be a successful writer, you should understand the process of publishing. If
you do this, you will know what is likely to happen to your manuscript and you
will also be better able to present your manuscript to maximise your chances
of being published.

Aims and scope of journal

In addition to reading the journal guidelines, you should investigate widely and
find the aims and scope of the journal you are submitting to. This will tell you
how the journal, that is, the publisher and editorial team, view their journal
and its purpose in relation to the kind of articles it wishes to publish. The aims
of journals tend to be very similar in terms of being international, exchanging
views, promoting scholarship and so on, but you need to ensure that you
address these, and the scope will tell you, for example, if the journal publishes
all types of research; for example, if it includes articles by midwifery and allied
health professions as well as nursing. If you are in any doubt, correspond
with the journal editorial office. For examples of the aims and scope (slightly
modified here) of two journals (*Journal of Clinical Nursing* and *Nurse Education
in Practice*), see Box 2.8; can you see how these differ and can you match the
aims and scope to these titles? If in doubt, check the journals online.

Box 2.8 Journal aims and scope

Journal 1

The journal is an international, peer-reviewed, scientific journal that
seeks to promote the development and exchange of knowledge that is
directly relevant to all spheres of nursing and midwifery practice. The
primary aim is to promote a high standard of clinically related scholarship that supports the practice and discipline of nursing. The journal
publishes high-quality manuscripts on issues related to clinical nursing,
regardless of where care is provided. This includes – but is not limited

to - ambulatory care, community care, family care, home, hospital, practice, primary and secondary and public health.

The journal also aims to promote the international exchange of ideas and experience that draws from the different cultures in which practice takes place. Further, the journal seeks to enrich insight into clinical need and the implications for nursing intervention and models of service delivery. An emphasis is placed on promoting critical debate on the art and science of nursing practice.

The journal endeavours to attract a wide readership that embraces experienced clinical nurses, student nurses and those who support, inform and investigate nursing practice. The development of clinical practice and the changing patterns of inter-professional working are also central to the journal's scope of interest. As such, contributions are welcomed from other health professions on issues that have a direct impact on nursing practice.

Journal 2

The journal enables lecturers and practitioners to both share and disseminate evidence that demonstrates the actual practice of education as it is experienced in the realities of their respective work environments, that is, both in the university/faculty and clinical settings. It is supportive of new authors and is at the forefront in publishing individual and collaborative manuscripts that demonstrate the link between education and practice.

Nursing is a discipline that is grounded in its practice origins - nurse educators utilise research-based evidence to promote good practice in education in all its fields. A strength of this journal is that it seeks to promote the development of a body of evidence to underpin the foundation of nurse education practice, as well as promoting and publishing education-focused manuscripts from other healthcare professions that have the same underpinning philosophy.

Case studies and innovative developments that demonstrate how nursing and healthcare educators teach and facilitate learning, together with reflection and action that seeks to transform their professional practice, will be promoted.

The opportunity to stimulate debate is encouraged as is the promotion of evidence-based nursing education internationally.

Editors and editorial board

All journals will have these; there will be a lead editor, sometimes called the editor or the editor-in-chief, depending on how the journal is managed. Both the editors of this book, like some of the chapter authors, are actually editors of international journals. The editor/editor-in-chief is the person employed by the publisher to run the journal on a day-to-day basis and, with the publisher, to set the policy and practice of the journal. Editors are usually established scholars in their own field. Editors are usually quite visible people nationally and internationally; they attend the key conferences in their field and it is good if you can make contact with them. They also give presentations on their journal, or workshops on how to submit to their journal. If you get the opportunity, attend these and gain a better understanding of how their journals function and what kind of articles are submitted. The work of editors and publishers is considered in Chapter 11.

Impact factor

An increasing number of journals have an impact factor, which is a measure of how often the articles published in the journal have been referred to (cited) by other authors in journals that, likewise, have an impact factor. The main system is operated by Thomson Reuters (http://tiny.cc/r9k49; Accessed 14 May 2011).

Impact factors are controversial and will not be discussed here at length but, to some extent, publishers judge the success of their journals by the impact factor as there is an annual ranking of journals by impact factor – a league table, if you like. Therefore, regardless of your views on impact factors you should realise that these are important to editors and publishers, and articles that are more likely to help a journal increase its impact factor are more likely, but by no means exclusively, to be published. There are other systems for tracking citations, and Scopus (http://www.scopus.com/home.url), which is the system operated by Elsevier, uses a tool called SCImago (www.scimagojr.com) to produce its own impact factors.

What increases impact factor?

Publishers are well aware of which articles increase impact factors and they study the performance of particular articles and types of manuscripts annually and share this information with their editors. The main manuscripts that contribute to impact factor are review manuscripts. These have always been important for journals because anyone investigating a new field will 'gravitate' towards review manuscripts (either titled Systematic or Literature Review); these are especially liked by research students who are likely to cite relevant reviews in their theses and subsequent publications. They are also a ready-made data set of prepared references that they can use as a source of material in their own searches!

In addition, review manuscripts have increased in importance and popularity with the advent of evidence-based practice and the refinement of review methods. Therefore, if you submit a review manuscript to a journal you increase your chances of being published. For examples of highly cited review manuscripts from *Journal of Clinical Nursing*, see Ross (2006) and Shields et al. (2006).

Other manuscripts that are known to increase the impact factor – and often for the same reasons as review manuscripts – are those focusing on research methodology, for example Rattray and Jones (2007). These manuscripts may be reviews of the use of methods or they may be manuscripts on the application of a new method or the introduction of a new method. Discursive manuscripts are known to increase impact factor as they often become 'turning points' in their field and, therefore, highly cited and a good example here is Paley (2001). Finally, outside of the aforementioned categories are miscellaneous topics manuscripts that become highly cited, and the reasons for this are hard to specify; usually, they are very high quality manuscripts by high-profile academics, but not always. Often, they address growing trends in the field or areas that are prioritised by governments for research funding.

What happens next?

Having considered getting started and the issues to consider in setting out on your writing journey, what you may ask happens next? As you will realise, every submission does not result in acceptance. However, many do thanks to good planning and effective writing strategies and this initiates another process of finally editing the manuscript to get the presentation up to the standards that the editor expects before it is sent to production. The process of publication is covered in Chapter 11. I hope that this chapter has helped you to begin that writing for publication experience and to have the confidence to 'have a go' at what is or can be a very rewarding personal and professional experience.

References

Hodson, P. cited in Swain, H. (2007) The write stuff and how to get it Times Higher Education 14 September. Available at: http://tiny.cc/h0ry7 [Accessed 14 May 2011].

King, S. (2004) Stephen king's advice for writers: read a lot; write a lot. Available at: http://tiny.cc/lsum8 [Accessed 14 May 2011].

Miser, H.J. (1998) Journal editing as I see it. *CBE Views*, 22, 71-75.

Paley, J. (2001) An archaeology of caring knowledge. *Journal of Advanced Nursing*, 36, 188-198.

Rattray, J. & Jones, M.C. (2007) Essential elements of questionnaire design and development. *Journal of Clinical Nursing*, 16, 234-243.

Ross, L. (2006) Spiritual care in nursing: an overview of the research to date. *Journal of Clinical Nursing*, 15, 852-862.

Russell, M. (2010) The independent climate change e-mails review. Available at: http://tiny.cc/dkxyo [Accessed 11 May 2011].

Salwak, D. (2011) Listen to your sentences. *Times Higher Education*, 7 (April), 44-47.

Shields, L., Pratt, J. & Hunter, J. (2006) Family centred care: a review of qualitative studies. *Journal of Clinical Nursing*, 15, 1317–1323.

Sullivan, E. (2002) Top 10 reasons a manuscript is rejected. *Journal of Professional Nursing*, 18, 1–2.

Watson, R. (2006) Writing an abstract. *Nurse Author & Editor* 16, 4. Available at: http://tiny.cc/nqqde [Accessed 11 May 2011].

Watson, R. (2011) Rules of writing for publication. Available at: http://tiny.cc/qtv4c [Accessed 11 May 2011].

Chapter 3

Writing a Conference Abstract and Paper

Jan Draper

Department of Nursing, Faculty of Health and Social Care, The Open University, Milton Keynes, UK

Introduction

The aim of this chapter is to provide guidance on how to write a successful conference abstract and conference paper. Whether you have previous experience or whether you are a complete novice, your first goal is to maximise the chances of your abstract being accepted. Your second goal, once accepted, is to write and present a high-quality conference paper.

What is the purpose of an abstract? The abstract gets you to the conference and, once there, gets delegates to your session. It should have a story that is worth hearing and that 'beats the competition'. Abstracts are, therefore, important, but they can be difficult to write because condensing the essence of something into a few words is harder than writing copious amounts. Distilling all you want to convey in the space of a word-limited abstract is a real skill; do not underestimate the difficulty.

> ### Activity 1
>
> If you have already had experience of writing an abstract, reflect on this experience. What was most rewarding? What did you find most difficult? If you have not yet written an abstract, imagine yourself at the starting line and ask what might be most rewarding and most challenging.

Perhaps the most rewarding aspect is the achievement of having your abstract accepted. Some of the challenges you identified might include the following:

Writing for Publication in Nursing and Healthcare: Getting It Right, First Edition.
Edited by Karen Holland and Roger Watson.

- Getting started.
- Sticking to the word count.
- Coming up with a title that grabs attention, is punchy and is informative.
- Achieving a logical flow and structure.
- Having the courage to acknowledge any limitations of your project.
- Not getting a rejection.

This chapter covers all these issues and is organised into two main sections: the first deals with how to write an abstract and the second with how to write and present a conference paper.

Section 1: How to write an abstract

What are the features of a good abstract?

Activity 2

Think back to a conference you have recently attended. Search out the conference pack, look through the abstracts and select one to review that you like. What are the features that you think make this a good abstract? What is it that you like about it? What is the pulling power? What grips?

When I used this activity at a conference workshop on how to write abstracts (Draper, 2009), participants identified the following features they like to see in an abstract:

- Relevance to the person reading.
- Use of short paragraphs.
- One that makes sense.
- A clear title, and one that is attention grabbing and has pulling power.
- The importance of the first paragraph.
- Clear headings so that the abstract is easily scanned.
- Outcomes that are honest.
- References that are kept to a minimum.
- A clear link between the ending and the beginning.
- A clear relationship between the title and what follows.
- A clear context and rationale – to understand the why and the what.
- Identification of questions and issues.
- Learning outcomes (depending on guidance).
- Careful use of bullet points.

Box 3.1 The features of a good abstract

- Audience
- Well written
- Concise and succinct
- No hidden assumptions
- Critical friend
- Engaging, catchy, open and inviting
- Attractive
- Your shop window, and opportunity to impress

- Follows guidance
- Convinces you can deliver
- Confident, authoritative style
- Attends to detail
- Consistent tense
- Careful use of abbreviations
- Sandwich technique

You might have identified similar features too and in Box 3.1, I have identified these along with others I also think are important. In the discussion that follows we will expand on these features.

Audience

Always make sure that you do your homework so that you know what type of conference it is, who the audience are and whether there will be international delegates. If so, then you will have to make sure that your language and style embrace a style that is not UK-centric or styled in a way that is mainly for the country you are from if not the United Kingdom. If it is an education conference you must make it educationally relevant. If it is a research conference, a focus on methodology and method is likely to be more appropriate. And if it is a conference about practice, your abstract will need to identify applications to and implications for practice. Think about who you would want to read your abstract and attend your presentation and tailor your abstract accordingly.

Well written

It is perhaps obvious to state the importance of ensuring your abstract is well written, but many are not. Work back from the submission deadline and take time to draft and re-draft. Always be concise, precise and succinct or as some colleagues will say – do not 'waffle' (meaning make pointless or irrelevant comments). Be extremely efficient with your use of words and continuously ask yourself 'do I need this word?' or 'will the meaning alter if I remove this word?' As with any writing, editing is crucial (see Chapter 2). Be careful to ensure you spell out at the beginning any assumptions you have made so that your context and position are clear. If this is not done, reviewers will assume that you are blind to these assumptions and may reject your abstract outright. Ask someone who does not know your work to act as a critical friend, to read through your abstract and to make sure that they can understand what it is you are trying to say.

Engaging and attractive

In addition to being well written, your writing style has to be engaging and inviting. But there is a need to be cautious here so that you do not become 'chatty' (informal kind of language) and overfamiliar. Your writing needs to be attractive and provide the 'grab' factor or something that will immediately get your attention. In this respect, the abstract title is crucial. The title needs to capture the topic accurately and link to what follows. It should not be too long or too short, and should create a sense of interest or intrigue (Fowler, 2011) while not being too obscure (Coad and Devitt, 2005). It should clearly articulate what you did, what you found and what your findings mean (Pierson, 2004).

Your shop window

Remember that the abstract is your 'shop window', your only opportunity at this stage to impress the reviewers with your work, to show them what you have done. Take this opportunity seriously and maximise your chances. Once through this stage, your challenge is then to continue to impress the delegates and entice them to come to your session at the conference. Your abstract will be published in the conference proceedings or even on the conference website and, once there, it remains the only vehicle to impress or direct delegates to want to attend your presentation at a conference, so it is worth carefully investing in your abstract preparation.

Conference guidance

Always follow the conference guidelines on how to submit an abstract – follow them closely. Different conferences have different approaches: some have very structured guidance, including instructions about layout, while others might only specify a word limit. Take time at the start to familiarise yourself with the guidance and make sure you follow it exactly. If the conference has several themes, be sure to identify to which theme you would like your abstract to align. For popular conferences where reviewers are inundated with abstract submissions, their decisions may come down to whether writers have adhered to the minutiae of the guidance so it is in your interests to follow the guidance carefully.

An example of broad criteria expectations regarding submission to a particular conference theme can be seen in the following guidance for submission of an abstract to the NETNEP 2012, 4th International Nurse Education conference (http://www.netnep-conference.elsevier.com/abstractsubmission.asp).

NETNEP 2012: consider the focus of each theme to select your abstract choice:

(1) *Continuing professional development/education*: The abstracts in this theme should reflect research, development and innovation, policy and practice in the continuing professional development (CPD) (life-long learning) of qualified nurses and midwives or career development for student

nurses and midwives preparing to become qualified nurses. This can include CPD/continuing professional education (CPE) developments such as short courses of study, postgraduate Master's level study or Doctoral level programs (PhD/Professional Doctorates).

(2) *Teaching, assessment and learning in University and clinical practice*: The abstracts in this theme should focus on any aspect of teaching, learning and assessment of students in both a practice and university context. This could relate to either a specific focus on the student experience itself or the role of faculty/lecturers and practice educators in this experience. It could also include the role of service users and carers/patients in the student learning experience.

(3) *Technology, simulation and education*: The abstracts in this theme should focus on the use of technology in its broadest context to enhance the student learning experience. This includes the use of technology in clinical simulation development and faculty/university clinical laboratories, as well as information literacy and technology.

(4) *Faculty and practice partnerships*: The abstracts in this theme should focus on partnerships between faculty and university and practice in a wide context, including the development of multi-disciplinary developments and working collaboratively to enhance all nursing and midwifery education programmes and professional development.

(5) *Research for education, policy and global developments*: The abstracts in this theme should focus on strategic evidence of where research-based evidence is making a significance to local, national and international developments and policy setting. Education for healthcare where research has made a difference is such an example, as is an inter-disciplinary and/or inter-professional context. Abstracts focusing on theoretical, historical or methodological approaches that promote discussion are welcomed.

More specific guidance for submission can be seen in Box 3.2.

A style that convinces you can deliver

The style, structure, content and tone you adopt in your abstract have to communicate to reviewers that you can deliver a good presentation. How you bring all these components together in a convincing way is essential to your success in abstract acceptance. Remember that the abstract summarises a paper that can be realistically delivered in 20 minutes, so it is important that you do not include too much information that you propose to deliver, as you will be unable to do so due to time factors. Less is definitely more when it comes to a conference presentation. As you draft the abstract, try to put yourself in the position of a reviewer and ask yourself whether you would be convinced by this writer's ability to deliver. Your abstract has to convince the reviewers that you can deliver and adopting a confident and authoritative style is crucial.

Box 3.2 Guidance for submission of a conference abstract: section A – oral (paper) presentation (with permission from NETNEP 2012 conference team (Elsevier))

- Oral (paper) sessions allow authors to present papers for discussion, detailing their latest research, education innovations and/or practice as educators.
- Oral (paper) sessions involve authors presenting for 20 minutes, with 10 minutes allocated for discussion. All submissions are subject to a double-blind peer-review process undertaken by members of the International Scientific Committee. The submission requirements are as follows:
  - Identification of relevant NETNEP theme(s) to which submitted (see Appendix 1).
  - Written in English. Font: Times New Roman, size 10; Harvard Reference style.
  - The title should be as brief as possible but long enough to indicate clearly the nature of the study. Capitalise the first letter of each word (except conjunctions). No full stop at the end.
  - An abstract of between 400–500 words (plus between 2–5 references to support the evidence base of the abstract content) is required (any abstract that exceeds the required word count will not enter the review process).
  - The abstract is required to include details of research, development and/or innovation, with sufficient information to enable the review panel to make a decision on appropriateness for oral presentation in theme and context of the conference (any research reported MUST have commenced at the time of the abstract submission).
  - Abstracts should state briefly and clearly the purpose, methods, results and conclusions/discussions of the work.
  - Key contact to be named and identified if there is more than one presenter of an oral paper.

Attention to detail

As we have already seen in other chapters of this book, attention to detail is important in academic writing of all kinds and the conference abstract is no exception. Ensure that you pay attention to detail, that you are consistent with, for example, abbreviations, spelling, spaces, capitals and referencing style. Be consistent with your use of tenses. Many writers switch between tenses for no apparent reason; therefore, choose your tense and then stick to it.

Structure

In terms of structure, the 'sandwich' technique is helpful at the early drafting stage. Start out with a clear beginning, describing what it is you are going to do. Then provide the detail in the middle section and conclude by outlining the implications for practice or education or research, or all three (depending on the specific guidance and the type of conference). There are several suggestions for structure (see, for example, Alexandrov and Hennerici, 2007; Happell, 2008) but while it is important you choose a structure that is clear and logical, it is equally important to choose one with which you feel comfortable. Some suggested structures lend themselves more to reporting empirical projects; however, abstracts do not always have to report empirical projects, they can be more theoretical or discursive. In this case it is important that you try not to squeeze your abstract into an ill-fitting structure; make sure you select one that best fits what you are trying to achieve. If you use headings or bullet points, do so carefully.

In summary, a good abstract is one that focuses on an interesting and topical issue, fits well with the themes of the conference and is therefore likely to be interesting to the expected audience. It is well presented and clearly argued, shows good awareness of the literature and is the right length for a conference paper. Having outlined these key features of a good abstract, in the next section we consider some of the common pitfalls reviewers observe.

What are some of the common pitfalls?

Activity 3

Imagine you have been invited by the conference organisers to be a reviewer of submitted abstracts. You may have possibly 30 or more to review. What do you think might be some of the common pitfalls writers fall into?

You might have identified some of the following:

- Trying to be too clever and impressing the reviewer with complicated language.
- Lacking focus.
- Using inappropriate language, thereby increasing the chances of being excluded before the abstract is formally reviewed.
- Waffly (such as using six words when one word would suffice), jargonistic (using terms that may be appropriate for a specific audience but not for wider audience when it becomes meaningless), buzzwords (words that are common to a specific group, like a second language) or too technical/scientific.

Box 3.3 Some common pitfalls

- Poor presentation
- Poor structure
- Not right conference
- Poor expression/unclear
- Does not follow guidance
- Ignores critical and/or relevant literature/no references
- No context
- Lack of evidence
- Poor use of language

- Too descriptive
- Too localised information
- Research has got to be completed!
- Too big/too small
- 'Salami' slicing
- UK-centric
- No proofreading – with typographical errors, grammar errors

- Complex sentences.
- Not knowing the audience.
- No context or background.
- The title not reflecting the content of the abstract/presentation.
- Not being mindful of national/international audience.

I have identified these and others in Box 3.3. While many of the pitfalls are the reverse features of a good abstract it is worth discussing these further.

Poor presentation

Poor presentation and structure are common. These are things that should be so easy to get right. Sometimes the abstract might be well written but not suitable for the audience of this particular conference. This underlines the importance of being wise about which conferences you identify as potential venues for dissemination of your work and then 'doing your homework' in relation to the conference. If you have not been to that conference before, try to find someone you know who has or at least look carefully at the conference website. Identify any previous events as the conference may well be an annual or bi-annual event with abstracts from previous conferences available for you to see in the conference proceedings.

Badly written

Issues of poor expression, lack of clarity and focus and not adhering to the guidance are also frequent problems cited by reviewers, so make sure that your abstract does not fall into one of these categories. Take time to draft and re-draft and make sure you are not working right up to the deadlines set and putting yourself under undue pressure. You need to allow sufficient time for critical reading, editing and re-drafting.

No context

While space is at a premium, you do need to make sure that you give your audience sufficient context so that they can locate the relevance of your presentation. Make sure you include reference to key literature while also being mindful of the specific guidance. Context and an evidence base are both important and while you will not have much space to elaborate in detail, you will need to give sufficient information for the reviewers to have confidence that you know relevant seminal work and wider evidence. Some conference guidelines indicate the number of references expected in the abstract (see Box 3.2).

Poor use of language

Wise and authoritative use of language is important in any writing, but when your word limits are so small, as it is in abstract writing, your style and use of language become even more important. So make sure your use of English is as good as it can be (if English not your first language and the 'conference language' is English, have the abstract read and edited by an English language speaker). Being too descriptive (the 'I did this and then I did that' approach) is also to be avoided. The assessment of your critical friend will be invaluable here, as it is hard to remain objective oneself. As you are writing, you also need to ensure that you are communicating effectively the essence of your work. Will it mean that the reviewers and subsequently the conference delegates will want to know more? The reviewers will want to be convinced that you have got something interesting to say and that others will want to hear you and also stimulate discussion and sometimes debate. Therefore, you have to communicate what this 'essence' is or else you run the risk of being consigned to the group of abstracts that are too local in their approach, and that lose meaning to the majority of the possible conference audience.

Ensure you have communicated clearly what contribution your work has made, or can make to the subject/discipline area. This contribution does not have to be the generation of new knowledge, but it could be a new insight on a familiar concept, or a slightly different approach to a method, methodology or a different combination of methods or theory. One approach at the outset of your abstract drafting might be for you to consider all the issues that come into your mind when you start thinking about your project and work to be conveyed. Sometimes writing this down in a mind map or spider diagram can be extremely helpful and 'unlock' ideas and associations of which you might not previously have thought.

Research that is completed

If you intend to present on an empirical project, be sure that you will have had time to complete the project, or undertaken a significant part of the data collection activities! This might sound obvious and eminently sensible but author submissions do not always take cognisance of this. The panel of reviewers have to be convinced that there will be something for the conference presenter to share with the delegates and many conferences, because of lack of findings or similar issues, have now started to make it very clear as one of the criteria for acceptance, or at least indicate on some way that the project has started, for example through identifying a pilot study or gaining research ethics approval.

Size

In terms of size and intent, be sure that your abstract is not too big or too small but that it is just at the right length. When reading your abstract, this will be one thing of which the reviewers will be mindful. If your abstract promises the conference audience to share too many different things and its scope is just too broad, the reviewers will be suspicious about you being able to keep to time should you get to the conference. Take care to judge the scope of what is required carefully and do not try to do too much.

'Salami slicing'

You may think on seeing this heading, why is the author talking about food preparation?!

'Salami slicing' is a word that you may come across in the literature. For example, If you have previously presented on this topic or project before, you have to be especially careful not just to 'slice' your work into sections but keep using parts of the same in terms of ideas and so on, and running the risk of self-plagiarism. You will need to communicate what it is that is different about this presentation. It might be that you have presented data in a slightly different way, or that you have used a different theoretical framework, or that the focus of the presentation is targeted in a slightly different way; for example that it has a policy rather than a practice focus. It is not good practice, in either writing an abstract or writing an article, to keep presenting work that has been used in multiple different ways, as it can cause readers and reviewers to think *'this person does not have anything new to share with us on this topic, and I heard them present this 3 years ago, but not much has moved on with their work'.*

Country specific focused (e.g. UK centric, Australia centric, US centric)

For those conferences aiming to attract international delegates, a frequent criticism of reviewers is that abstracts are often chosen that represent the host country's language and developments. At one end of the spectrum, this can relate merely to careless use of local language, abbreviations and terminology. This is relatively easy to rectify.

At the other end of the spectrum it can mean that the focus of the whole abstract is so country specific focused that it does not provide any potential for drawing out implications for a wider international context. For example it is possible for any parochial local-based project to be communicated or 'branded' in such a way that it has potential relevance to an international audience. Things to bear in mind are as follows:

- Take care not to use abbreviations. For example, instead of using 'NMC' (Nursing and Midwifery Council) use a broad term that would be understood by the international audience, such as 'professional regulatory body'.
- When setting the context, do not just think, for example 'United Kingdom' 'United States' or 'Japan', but think wider. So rather than writing something like 'Research evidence suggests...' write 'Research evidence in the United Kingdom and the wider international community suggests...' This is also good practice for writing full articles (see Chapter 5).
- When identifying implications for practice, education, management or research, remember these need to embrace a wider international community, so you can allude to the fact that you will identify these in your presentation.

Proofreading

Careful proofreading is one of the most important stages of the whole process, as it is for any writing activity where someone else is going to be reading and reviewing it. First, proofread the abstract yourself to ascertain if you have incorporated all the issues identified previously and then, second, get someone else to read it for you. Ask them to look at it as if they knew nothing about the subject. Does it make sense? Does it flow? Is it coherent? Does it do what it says it will do? Does it have internal consistency? Does it tick all the boxes of the 'features of a good abstract' (see Box 3.1)?

Summary

Once you have finalised all your preparatory work and are completely satisfied that your abstract is as complete as it can be, that it has followed all the conference guidance, you are ready to submit to the conference organisers. Make sure you follow this submission guidance carefully and ensure that you submit everything on time! Once submitted, all you can do is wait and, in anticipation of acceptance, begin to think about preparing your presentation, which may or may not be accompanied by a short conference paper to be included in the proceedings book.

Section 2: How to write a conference presentation

You hear good news that your submitted abstract has been accepted for the conference and that you are expected to prepare a presentation and, along with that, some kind of informative paper for the delegate.

Having got your abstract accepted and written in such a way that it has caught the attention of the reviewers who believe that it will attract lots of delegates to your session, how then do you write a great paper that delivers all it promises? Often, at conferences we are attracted by abstracts in the conference proceedings and, unfortunately, the actual paper or presentation of what the abstract has told us about your work turns out to be a real disappointment. So, how can you avoid this and make sure your paper lives up to its expectations?

Activity 4

Think back to a really bad conference presentation you attended. What was it that made it so bad? Was it content, the way it was delivered or both?

We easily remember the bad conference presentations we have attended rather than those we have enjoyed! Some of the aspects of a bad presentation you identified might have included the following:

- Poor time keeping by the presenter.
- Presenter too quiet when presenting the work or sits there and reads from a scripted sheet of paper.
- No setting of context explained to the delegates.
- Unclear storyline and structure.
- Imbalance between different sections of the presentation when the abstract promises more.
- Too much information on the slides.
- Just reading from slides.
- Typographical/grammatical errors on the slides.
- Poor or inconsistent presentation on slides.
- Country-centric acronyms.
- Recommendations that are too big and unrealistic.
- Patronising style of presentation, that is talking to the audience as if you know everything and they do not – saying it in a way that makes this very clear and is very apparent to the audience, the presenter appears to have no respect for the audience's intellect or understanding of the topic and issues being presented.

Therefore, how can we learn from our own and others' past mistakes to ensure that in the future all our conference papers are of really high quality? It is one thing to prepare a conference paper/presentation, it is another to deliver it in a professional and engaging way, and in this final section of the chapter we consider some top tips for both.

Preparing your paper

In making your preparations for the presentation, you need to decide how you are going to deliver it on the day, as the actual style of delivery should inform the way you prepare. For example if you intend to have very detailed notes in front of you from which to read, you will have to prepare these in advance along with the slides. If your planned style is rather more informal and spontaneous, you may wish to have bullet points in front of you but you will still have to make sure that you are able to broaden out or expand on these bullet points on the day. It is crucial to have decided on your delivery style so that your preparations are made accordingly, personal preference and the nature of the conference should inform this decision. If, for example, the conference is large and international, you may be more likely to opt for a formal scripted approach. If it is a smaller conference, you may feel a slightly less formal presentation would be more suitable. Doing your homework about the conference, its expectations of presenters and time allowed for them is, therefore, very important.

There are several factors to consider as you prepare your paper/presentation, including audience, timing, content and structure, audiovisual aids and delivery style. These are also aspects you will need to bear in mind when you come to deliver your paper and we will consider each of them in turn. It is important to note here that we often talk about the 'delivery of a paper' at a conference. What we mean by this is, in reality, the delivery of an oral presentation that can or may be supported by an actual written paper outlining the core elements of the work to be presented. This is often used for many presenters as a testing out of ideas and thoughts for an actual article for publication at a later stage (see Chapter 9).

Delivery of the conference paper

Audience

Detailed information about the audience is important in preparing the abstract; remembering to keep your audience in mind as you prepare the paper is also important. Think about who this audience is, who they are likely to be and what aspects of your work they may be particularly interested in. Given the nature of the conference, are they likely to be practitioners, researchers, educationalists or a mixture? The constituency of delegates should, therefore, inform the way you balance the writing of your paper and the actual presentation of it.

Timing

To ensure you remain within your allotted time, you must ensure that your paper is not too long. You are likely to have a maximum of 20 minutes to deliver your paper (presentation of what it is you have included in your abstract plus more detailed aspects of the work) and it is surprising how quickly 20 minutes can disappear. Some conferences will then allow 5 minutes for questions while others might expect questions to be taken within the 20-minute allocation. It is, therefore, important to establish exactly how much time you have by carefully consulting the conference guidance. If necessary, seek additional information from the conference organisers.

Achieving a balance between the different components of your presentation is crucial; a common mistake is for the context-setting/background or the literature overview to take too long. This then means there is less time to devote to the real essence of your paper. A good conference chairperson will ensure all presenters keep to time, so to have a 5-minute warning that your session is nearly over when you feel you have only just begun is incredibly distracting! You might wish to agree with the chairperson for your presentation session some other arrangement depending on the way you wish to present the work.

Therefore, take time to think carefully about the breakdown of the various components of your presentation. Always anticipate your delivery will take longer on the day – because it will! If you have 20 minutes (plus 5 or 10 minutes then for questions/discussion) and your presentation is about a project (as opposed to something more theoretical or developmental) you might wish to consider the following approach. Establishing this outline at the start of your preparations is important as it gives an immediate guide to the relative balance of the different components of the presentation and where you should be directing your efforts.

Content and structure

Adopting a clear and logical structure and developing a coherent storyline that takes your audience along with you are crucial to your success in presenting what you intended. It is also important to achieve continuity between the abstract and the actual paper, to ensure that your paper delivers what the abstract said it would. It may be a few months since you submitted your abstract; enough time for you to forget the details, so always have your abstract beside you to remind you of what you said you would say.

Depending on whether you have already established preferences, there are several approaches to preparing your presentation. You can work on the full-scripted paper first, which for some of you at this time may be in note form or if you have been asked to also provide a more structured evidence-based conference paper as well, the audience may already be able to access this in the conference proceedings book or as a separate supplement. Some conferences invite authors to submit their work as a core paper, which is then linked to a group of papers around the same topic. You can then prepare accompanying slides or you can begin working on the slides first and then develop the accompanying paper or notes.

At the beginning of your paper, it is important to state the purpose of the paper clearly and its relevance to the conference themes. You should be able to draw on the abstract to inform this. Next you should signpost the overarching structure of the presentation, which can be achieved very concisely with a slide. The headings on this slide then need to feed through into the main presentation. It can be easy to present more in this context-setting or background, as in your enthusiasm you will want to get across to the audience the importance of undertaking the project or development, so take care not to digress too much from what you have in your presentation slide and accompanying notes, but stick to the point – advice that will be reiterated several times in the rest of this chapter.

You then need to set up the context and rationale for why you did this project. This might be because it was part of an undergraduate or postgraduate programme of study, or perhaps was an externally funded project, or a project undertaken as an organisational objective. Giving a context is important as it helps the audience understand where you are coming from. But again, be precise and stick to the point.

In the context of the project's rationale, reference to its location with respect to the relevant literature is important. What is the current evidence base about this particular issue? What might be some of the limitations of this evidence base? Are there gaps in knowledge? Are there any methodological limitations you wish to expose? Establishing at the beginning of the presentation why there was a need to do your project then provides a clear route back in towards the end, to conclude whether the project achieved what it set out to do.

You then need to outline your methodology and methods, taking care to provide a rationale for all your decisions. If, for example, you adopted an ethnographic methodology, be sure to explain why this was most appropriate for the project. Be concise in describing the research methods used, your sample and selection methods, issues related to ethical approval and methods of data analysis. The real key is to achieve a balance between too little and too much detail. The key is to maintain a focus as close to the purpose outlined in the abstract as possible; if it was the methodology then this is what the focus would be, if the findings and implications for practice then again the general how and why the project was undertaken would be kept brief in the presentation but may well be accompanied by a handout or a short written paper, accompanied by key literature. Some presenters also enable their presentation with contact details to be made available post-conference and others may submit their work to a journal for publication, either as a conference special issue or as a journal article (see Chapter 9).

The presentation of your findings should form the hub of the paper. It is likely that delegates will be most interested to hear what you found and will have come to your session explicitly for this purpose. You should devote proportionately more time to this section, so make sure that your timings reflect this (Box 3.4). As you prepare, identify the key findings. What are the headlines? If you had 2 minutes to describe to someone what you had found, what would you say? If you adopted a methodology that generated qualitative data, illustrating your key findings with excerpts from these data is always helpful and brings findings to life. If you are drawing on quantitative data, illustrate your findings with careful use of quantitative data presentation methods. Take care not to have too many tables or bar charts and pie charts.

In your concluding comments you should extract what you think are the key messages for the conference community and what you consider to be the implications for practice, education or research, or all three. Were there key findings that surprised you or aspects of the methodology or methods that you found interesting? Remember, it is not always just the data that might be

> **Box 3.4** Example presentation time allocation and content (project)
>
> Purpose of the paper *1 minute*
> Signposting of structure *1 minute*
> Context/rationale for the project *2 minutes*
> Location within existing literature *3 minutes*
> Brief outline of approach, methodology and methods *4 minutes*
> Summary of key findings *6 minutes*
> Conclusions and implications for practice, education or research *3 minutes*

interesting for delegates but also any analysis of the utility of the methodology and methods or the theoretical framework you used.

Audiovisual aids

Visual slides using a programme such as Microsoft PowerPoint help to illustrate the presentation and provide visual anchors for the audience to communicate key messages and signpost structure. They will help you to help your audience understand and remember your presentation. Depending on the conference, printed copies are often made available for the audience either during the actual presentation or afterwards. If available during the presentation, they can help to focus audience attention and if provided afterwards, become a physical reminder of your presentation. Slides are, therefore, a central component of your conference presentation and it is crucially important to carefully prepare your slide presentation (Box 3.5).

If you want some dialogue with the audience (dependent on the nature of the conference), for example to get their views on a particular aspect of your work, be sure to build this in to your presentation. This can be done by including a final slide with particular questions to prompt discussion or thoughts about audience feedback. It is also helpful to provide your email address on this final slide so delegates can get back in touch with you after the conference, if they want to.

Delivering your paper

You have now arrived at the conference and have to prepare for your presentation as well as actually attending the conference itself and listen to and support other presenters, maybe even colleagues from your own workplace. Make sure that you have back up copies of the presentation, any papers or handouts to the audience with you, as well as ensure that a copy of the presentation has been sent to the conference organisers, as is often a requirement

Box 3.5   Top tips for a PowerPoint presentation

Adopt a consistent design style throughout.

Do not let your choice of presentation design take precedence, overtake your presentation content and restrict your message.

Chose an easy-to-read font that is of a size that the audience can see.

Use consistent font sizes for headings and text.

Be careful with your use of colour and ensure that all colours are easy on the eye.

Decorate sparingly, that is not too many additional extraneous material, such as photos, artwork or interactive data (unless of course it is linked to the project explanation).

Do not put too much information on each slide. Leave some space.

Keep your information simple. Stick to key words, not sentences.

Slides should summarise the storyline and not become it.

Never read from your slides. They are not your script and are there to support not replace your talk.

Use animations and slide transitions very carefully. Too much 'whiz and bang' is distracting.

Practice presenting with your slides. Know them well.

Do not be tempted to have too many.

for many conferences. Make sure that you have had confirmation of receipt of this if this has been a conference policy.

Delivery style

We have already noted the importance of thinking ahead about your delivery style and how this should have informed the preparations for your paper. So, whatever your style of delivery make sure you practice beforehand. This is very important. Practice your verbal delivery and the style and the timing. You should speak to the audience, not to the slides, so you will need to look up from notes to give eye contact to the audience. Remember to speak clearly and loudly enough and not too fast. Being able to easily read your notes while presenting is important and a useful tip is to use a larger than normal font size for the print out of your notes. This will help prevent you getting lost as you look up and down, from your notes to the audience. Engaging with the audience, through eye contact, careful use of humour and a skilful oral style will be crucial to the success in the delivery of your paper. Gaining their confidence through an authoritative style is key to your success. This also applies to the ever-increasing practice at many conferences whereby delegates are invited to present in the same way but for a much shorter time (e.g. 5 minutes) as a poster presenter, whereby the main ideas presented in visual images and language are discussed with delegates.

In addition to practicing your delivery in whatever time limit, also practice how you are going to manage the presentation itself. You could use a mouse, keyboard or handheld device, and often the room layout will influence this choice. So always visit the room you will be presenting in beforehand to check the layout, the positioning of the laptop, where you can put your notes and where you will stand. It is good to have made all these decisions before you get up to speak so that there are no surprises on the day. If making an oral presentation of your poster, always try and ensure that not only are handouts available at the time, but are also made available to delegates at allocated poster viewing times when an oral presentation is not possible. This increases the opportunities for further dialogue with colleagues during the conference. For many colleagues new to presenting a paper at a conference this can provide a valuable opportunity to gain confidence in talking and sharing ideas about your work with peers but in much smaller numbers, which is less threatening in terms of being nervous or worried about talking in front of large groups.

Summary

If you have done all of this you are now ready to stand up and deliver your presentation. With meticulous preparation you can enter the conference session with confidence, knowing that you have done everything you can to feel prepared. All that remains is for you to enjoy the experience.

Well, almost! Once your presentation is over, it is always beneficial to seek out any evaluation of your session. The conference organisers are likely to have a formal post-conference evaluation questionnaire. It is worthwhile ensuring that you ask them for the evaluation data on your particular presentation. It is sometimes also helpful to seek out a friendly delegate and ask them for some informal feedback. All of this can provide helpful indicators for how you can improve your conference presentations in the future.

If you have provided a written paper for the presentation session, it is also important to continue with its development into an article for publication, to give more people an opportunity to read about your work and also to enhance your experience of publishing further. Writing that all-important abstract is the key to successful acceptance at a conference, not only as an oral presentation but also as the alternative of a poster presentation, which is a different media for dissemination of your work. It is hoped that the tips and content of this chapter will give you the confidence to submit a quality abstract and have it accepted at your chosen conference. Subsequently, other chapters in this book will give you added support and guidance to further develop that presentation and initial paper into a published paper (Chapters 9 and 5). Dissemination of research and practice development (see Chapter 15) in any field is essential for the progression of the scholarly community in any discipline and your oral presentation of your successful abstract is but the first stage on this all important journey.

References

Alexandrov, A.V. & Hennerici, M.G. (2007) Writing good abstracts. *Cerebrovascular Diseases*, 23(4), 256-259.

Coad, J. & Devitt, P. (2005) Research dissemination: the art of writing an abstract for conferences. *Nurse Education in Practice*, 6, 112-116.

Draper, J. (2009) *How to write an abstract.* Interactive workshop, Nurse Education Today Conference, 8-10 September, University of Cambridge, Cambridge, UK.

Fowler, J. (2011) Writing for professional publication. Part 11: writing conference abstracts. *British Journal of Nursing*, 20(7), 451.

Happell, B. (2008) Conference presentations: a guide to writing the abstract. *Nurse Researcher*, 15(4), 79-87.

Pierson, D.J. (2004) How to write an abstract that will be accepted for presentation at a national meeting. *Respiratory Care*, 49(10), 1206-1212.

Further reading

Coad, J., Devitt, P. & Hardicre, J. (2007) Ten steps to developing an abstract for conferences. *British Journal of Nursing*, 16(7), 396-397.

Happell, B. (2007) Hitting the target! A no tears approach to writing an abstract for a conference presentation. *International Journal of Mental Health Nursing*, 16, 447-452.

Hardicre, J., Coad, J. & Devitt, P. (2007) Ten steps to successful conference presentations. *British Journal of Nursing*, 16(7), 402-404.

Chapter 4

Writing for Publication: The Book Review

Dean Whitehead

School of Health and Social Services, Massey University, Palmerston North, Wellington, New Zealand

Introduction

Any form of academic writing constitutes an 'onerous' task for most health-care professionals – particularly fledgling writers, academics and researchers (Whitehead, 2000; Whitehead, 2002; Whitehead et al., 2007). Parker et al. (2010) agree and argue that academic writing is not a traditional part of nursing culture and, thus, never easy. Regan and Pietrobon (2010, p. 437) have also stated about academic writing:

> Despite its relevance to nursing, education about this essential skill is not currently evidence based and relies on a combination of mentorship and trial and error.

I do not recall any mentorship during my initial attempts to publish; but I do recall plenty of trial-and-error attempts, which gave me the feeling that there was some kind of 'pinnacle of great publishing' that I would need to reach and that seemed to thwart my attempts at every twist and turn.

Personal experience

My first experience of submitting for publication (some 15+ years ago) was not a great one and resulted in non-publication after a lengthy period of review and re-review. Thinking back now, it could have easily been my last attempt had I not been stubborn enough to want to prove those particular

Writing for Publication in Nursing and Healthcare: Getting It Right, First Edition.
Edited by Karen Holland and Roger Watson.
© 2012 John Wiley & Sons, Ltd. Published 2012 by John Wiley & Sons, Ltd.

editors wrong. Coming up to 100 international peer-reviewed journal articles later, I'm glad that I did not give up at that first hurdle. What does strike me, however, is that things are different today and perhaps it is a little easier to get started and, because there is more focus on the mentorship aspects and peer support, being able to find that first rung on the academic publishing ladder. Back in the time that I refer to, the opportunity to 'cut ones teeth' (test out one's early skills) so to speak or make that first attempt at writing of any kind was not as readily available as it is today. Book and other media reviews were not as visible in health professional journals, magazines and other related forums. Certainly, other more recent technological social media formats, that is web forums, weblogs, social blogs, wikis, tweets or podcasts that can assist writing today were certainly not available at all even a short while ago. Griffiths and Nicholls (2010), in their recent study, acknowledge rapidly changing technological environments and report their use of blogs and wikis to facilitate collaborative learning and writing.

There is no shortage of books and articles on the process of academic writing (Murray, 2009). There are also related books on 'how to' write PhDs, other types of thesis and research projects (Murray, 2002; Robson, 2007; Dunleavy, 2010). However, as might be expected, there is little by way of specific reference to writing book and media reviews outside of this text. A quick search on the Internet will unveil many anecdotal and often unstructured examples of writing media reviews, but none of them fulfil the requirements of a book chapter. It is hoped that this chapter provides a unique 'one-stop' resource for those contemplating writing media reviews.

What are the different types of media for review?

Most academic journals offer the facility of critically reviewing submitted full articles (mainly those that are primary research), but that is different to and beyond the scope of this chapter (see Chapter 5). Instead, what is referred to here is what might appear paradoxical; shorter reviews of longer pieces of work, that is books, theses, DVDs and other media types. For the purposes of this chapter, 'review' is used as a catch-all term that covers all these types of media. The most common form of media review, however, for publishing in academic journals is a book review – and many journals currently publish these as an important section of the journal along with the appointment of a Book Review Editor to oversee the work of a book review panel and monitor quality of the book review process. They also liaise with the publishers on book review evaluations and similar issues.

Not all journals have this facility and some that are currently doing so may well not pursue it in the future. If you feel that nursing-specific journals offer a limited option to publish in this format, Polit and Northam (2010) identify a large range of non-nursing journals (but which have direct relevance) that may also offer this facility.

Activity 1

Access a journal that currently publishes media reviews and has a Media Review Editor who oversees this process, for example *Nurse Education Today*, *Nurse Education in Practice*. How many other nursing or related health professional journals can you find that offer similar opportunities? Make a list of these and identify what their criteria are for becoming a book review panel member.

It is possible that in the not-too-distant future we will see the widespread acceptance and critical review of emerging and influential social media. These are media for social interaction that use highly accessible and scalable publishing techniques, particularly web-based technologies, that is blogs, twitters (Twitter) or Wikis. Currently, they tend to broadcast media monologues into broader social media dialogues – but detailed monologues that stand on their own (and are therefore reviewable) are becoming more common. Expanding technological conventions for media review offer potential authors ever-increasing options to see their work 'in print' or online.

Does writing a review differ from other scholarly publications?

The answer to this question of whether writing a review differs from writing other scholarly work is both yes and no. Yes, in terms of writing length, rigour of peer-review process (that is double-blind peer review, single peer reviewer or Media Review Editor review decision-making) and the time to publication. However, in most other aspects it is similar.

It is worth noting also that the convention for media reviews will mirror other relatively short academic journal submissions such as commentaries, letters and editorials (see Chapter 16). For shorter reviews, commentaries and so forth, it is expected that the author(s) will write in a structured academic style and therefore in a critical and objective manner. It is not unusual, for instance, for Review Editors to request critical debate within reviews by drawing on both comparative and contrasting or opposing literature. The conventions on correct citation style and reference list format apply as equally as they do to main articles in journals. Where this is the case, authors will need to be aware of the house-style convention, that is American Psychological Association (APA), American Medical Association (AMA), Vancouver (numerical), Harvard, Chicago, etc. (see Chapter 5 for in-depth explanation of these citation formats, style and conventions).

Failure to understand and comply with correct conventions such as referencing may equate to *the review/article being rejected*. As Hawkins (2009, p. 1) has stated:

> ... *the existence of several sets of guidelines for format and referencing can be enough to stifle any dreams of writing for publication.*

Activity 2

Following on from Activity 1, access again the journals you found that currently publish media reviews and have a Media Review Editor who oversees this process. What does the format look like? Does the structure, for example citation styles, differ between them – and how? Do you understand the different types of formats? If not, make a note to become familiar with them.

Why write book/media reviews?

Book/media reviews are often not only the easiest and quickest route to publication, but they also represent a very useful means for improving both writing and analytical skills; something that benefits both beginning and experienced writers. Both Nelms (2004) and Taylor et al. (2004) are quick to point out that writing for publication is important for the career development of nurses. Some go as far as to suggest that not writing for publication is 'unethical' (Savitz, 2000). Nurses generally write in one form or another most of their careers, yet there is a known and notable shortage of nurses who publicly write for publication (Keen, 2007).

For those who are taking the time and interest to read this chapter, the likelihood is that they have heard of or encountered the 'publish or perish' phenomenon (McGrail et al., 2006). For those who have not, this is a phrase used to make the point that, unless you publish anything at all it will end in poor career prospects for you, especially for those wishing to pursue career pathways in academia, especially at reader or professor level where there is an expectation of national and international focused publications.

Grympna (2007, p. 1) offers an anecdotal account of her first encounter with the concept of publish or perish, when attending a nursing-related interview and being unexpectedly asked 'what have you published and where?' She was relieved that, despite being a fledgling writer, she was able to offer at least some tentative examples. It was this particular encounter that introduced her to '... the implication that publications were the only measure of my academic worth'.

Leading on from this sentiment, what is known is that those who publish usually have the confidence and motivation to do so and, as a result, usually possess the momentum to continue writing. However, it is also worth bearing in mind that having written work accepted for publication is not an endpoint: it is merely the beginning or a platform for confidence and advancement. For those who have no publishing experience (and particularly students who are or have recently studied at both undergraduate and postgraduate levels), I would recommend looking to your 'best' last academic assignment/essay/report/thesis. It may give you the basis for structuring your writing for publication – but, to do so, you would need to compare and contrast such work against published

Table 4.1 Holland (2010 – adapted) guidelines for the 'general' review of a book.

(1) What does the title tell you about the book?

(2) When you are reading it does the title reflect accurately what the book includes? In other words, does the book meet your expectations of what the title states?

(3) Who are the authors?

(4) Is the book focused on national nursing programmes or is it a translated one?

(5) Who is the readership of the book? That is, is it aimed at undergraduate or postgraduate level students?

(6) If you are a student for whom the book is aimed at in terms of content and level, is it understandable to you? Are you able to read it easily?

(7) Does the book have additional supporting material that you can use? For example does it have a CD-ROM included as part of the book, to which you can refer to at different chapters or may have direct links to web-based resource?

(8) Does the book follow a logical sequence in terms of chapters?

(9) Is the content up-to-date with regard to supporting evidence or literature? Are these accessible should you wish to obtain them for reference?

(10) If there are illustrations, are these not too many to be distracting to you in relation to the content?

(11) How much does it cost? Is this good value when it comes to what the content is?

(12) Does the book have links to online material? This is a developing trend with publishers, to provide supporting material for students.

(13) As a student would you recommend it to others?

articles. Heyman and Cronon (2005) offer a useful guide to adapting academic work into publishable articles, as does Mark Hayter in Chapter 8 of this book. Holland (2010) also offers pertinent advice for students who wish to generally review books and write potential reviews of them. Table 4.1 denotes what this entails.

Other readers, but especially those studying or working in academic environments, will often be familiar with the requirements and rigours of publishing to attract individual and institutional funding. An example of this drive to publish to attract as much government funding for research as possible is seen in the Research Excellence Framework (REF) in the United Kingdom and the Performance Based Research Funding (PBRF) initiative in New Zealand (see 'Websites' at the end of the chapter for links to information about these very important publishing drivers).

For those who find the prospect of 'exposing' themselves to the scrutiny of peers and others, in the form of public writing, book and media reviews represent a valuable opportunity to get started. It is well highlighted that a lack of personal confidence and any questioning of ability to write are the main barriers preventing individuals from 'putting pen to paper' (Driscoll and Driscoll, 2002; Miracle, 2003; Heinrich et al., 2004). Also considered here, is

Box 4.1 Writing in action

Parker et al. (2010) report their Australian project, which had three main aims: (1) to build capacity in beginning writers, (2) to build capacity in beginning reviewers and (3) to produce a quality journal to celebrate local scholarship and research. They did this by developing a local co-funded journal for nurses and midwives called Handover, which was managed by an editorial committee consisting of experienced members from the area health service and two local universities. Two editions later, the authors were able to report a good degree of success, whereby novice writers were better motivated to submit their work for publication and where they also learnt to peer review others' work; assisting further with their writing skills and confidence. *The journal incorporated a variety of submission types – so submitting authors were able to test and hone their skills beginning with reviews.*

the additional academic writing barrier to those for whom English is a second language (Salamonson et al., 2009).

On the other hand, reviews also represent a convenient format for experienced authors who are 'time-pressured' to produce full articles but still want to maintain their writing profile. For experienced writers who find themselves in a 'writing lull' or 'block', they represent a useful platform for re-establishing momentum. They are good formats too for those experienced professionals and institutions that set up 'writing clubs' and other forms of peer-reviewed support groups when mentoring and supporting emerging writers. An excellent example of how practitioners developed their writing skills in collaboration with university colleagues can be seen in Box 4.1.

Whether reviewing a book through the auspices of a journal review panel or undertaking a book review for the publisher as part of your role as a clinician or lecturer when deciding on the recommended book list for students undertaking a programme of study, there is an additional benefit that you are able to keep the book or DVD as part of the review process.

Writing successful and effective book/media reviews

First and foremost, effective writing of any kind requires both adequate planning and attention to detail. All academic writing requires attention to due process and structure. With reviews this is no different, so always plan a structured course of action. As Silver (2009, p. 9) puts it very well *'writers don't plan to fail, but they often fail to plan'*. Remember also – a *book/media review* is not the same as a *book/media report*. The latter simply summarises the content presented.

While a review summarises to a certain extent, this is done far more critically – and other dimensions are reported on too. Most media reviews subsequently will follow a certain format. For instance, heading the review will usually be the book details as if it were a citation but with additional details such as number of pages, ISBN number (for ordering purposes) and recommended cost. The introductory paragraph will usually set the scene in terms of aims and objectives of the text. Subsequent paragraphs will usually denote, in sequence, an overview of the main contents of the text. Latter paragraphs will identify strengths and weaknesses of the text – with a concluding recommendation (or not) paragraph. Strengths and weaknesses should be written objectively (see later tips on effective writing). Many authors will naturally feel that it is less threatening to discuss strengths of others work than their weaknesses. Discussing weaknesses, however, is a natural part of a good review. Not all reviewed texts will be 'complete' and most are constrained by various factors – such as publishers word limit. Recommendations are best centred on issues such as what the information means in terms of the 'big picture', how the author(s) could expand on the results, what knowledge gaps might be evident and how the topic could be moved forward and expanded upon.

Nowadays, do remember that it is an increasingly common practice for published books to have accompanying support materials, that is CDs, CD-ROMs in the books and online links to such material, and more (such as Evolve with books published through Elsevier). Where this is the case, the expectation is that you would review this material as well and incorporate it to your critical review. Sometimes, although rarely, some publishers send out this type of material (mainly video/DVD) to review on its own. The conventions should be similar to constructing a book review – but check with the Review Editor first. In most cases, Review Editors prefer not to send out this type of material for review on its own, as it does not offer the reviewer of the material a total picture of the product and the accompanying book.

Tip 1

Initially 'skim and scan' the text to identify its main points. Reading from 'cover-to-cover' in one sitting is likely to lead to 'word fatigue'. As you read through, make notes that act as prompts for later writing of the whole review. Faigley (2011) also suggests reading and viewing with a 'critical eye', which involves the overall process of: preview; summarise, respond; and analyse.

Activity 3

Pick up any academically structured textbook (or other similar media) that is readily at hand to you in preparation for a 'mock' review. Then 'hypothetically' choose a journal that you have encountered in Activities 1 and 2 previously. Before you begin, what do you think are some of the things that you might need to consider for ensuring a smooth overall process?

Tips for writing effective book/media reviews: avoiding the pitfalls

As Heyman and Cronon (2005, p. 401) suggest:

> *Although writing skills at any level cannot be wholly taught, as their acquisition requires a combination of talent and development through practice, an element of early training can provide beginners with a tool kit that they can draw upon so as to avoid obvious pitfalls.*

This sentiment highlights the fact that effective writing skills are part of a 'tried-and-tested' process, which is already known to many. Acknowledging and acting upon this advice will save a lot of time, effort and disappointment. Before embarking on writing an academic review, take the time to digest the following points:

(1) Do you know what you are doing? If not, it is best not to pretend that you do. Even though writing reviews may not seem that demanding to those that have not done one before, it is a flawed assumption. As highlighted previously, for most nurses, many academic writing endeavours are neither natural nor easy. Keen (2007) highlights the main self-explanatory support strategies for novice writers, regardless of the type of the nature of the exercise. These being: attending credible academic writing courses, consulting publishing experts such as writing coaches, writing collaboratively with experts and seeking out peer-reviewed 'writing groups'. McVeigh et al. (2002) similarly highlight the merits of establishing and writing within 'publication syndicates', while Baldwin and Chandler (2002) further promote the merits of seeking out writing coaches. After all, scholarly publication is a social process and best avoided as an activity undertaken in isolation (Rhoads, 2006).

(2) Take it seriously, especially if you have been approached by a Journal Review Editor to write a review and join a panel of book and media reviewers. Do not see it as 'just a book review' and, therefore, not as important as an editorial, conference abstract or article. The Review Editor will not invite you again if you do not write the review or do not keep to deadlines agreed for its completion. More importantly still, if someone has read your review and subsequently bought the book (or not of course) based on your recommendation and then, on using it, asks themselves 'what is that person (reviewer) doing recommending this book?', then that can affect your credibility with the Review Editor as well as peers. Although there may be a degree of subjectivity in reviewing texts between different individuals, there should be a certain degree of overall 'consensus' as to what is good, bad and indifferent material. The Book and Media Editor will ensure of course that a review is constructive in its critique/summary and not destructive in its commentary prior to its publication. This does not mean, however, that perceived drawbacks with that being reviewed will

not be published. As with peer-reviewed articles (see Chapter 5) the editor may ask you to revise the review prior to final acceptance.

(3) As with all academic literature, nothing is 'perfect'. Personally I have only ever reviewed one book where my comments were far more on the positive side than anything else. It was a book that had nothing to do with my area of expertise or interest (a book on working in theatre recovery rooms). The fact that it caught my attention from the first cursory glance was essentially down to the fact that it was very well written, its' content was interesting and easy to follow, could be read in sections rather than in its totality to be able to understand the content and it did what it said it did; no more or less than that. That said, I still found one or two things to improve on and offered some constructive comments. These book reviews are taken seriously by publishers as they also help in the development of subsequent new editions of the book. Publishers engage reviewers to undertake this kind of review also when authors submit book proposals and the publisher needs to be assured that there is a need for the book and that the people who are proposing it will be able to deliver the manuscript within an agreed timeline.

(4) When asked to review a certain book it is important to determine if there is also any conflict of interest in undertaking the book review. For example it could be as simple as review of a book written by a work colleague or as complicated as reviewing a book that a relative has written! It is important to let the Book Review Editor know as soon as possible that you have this connection and that you do not think it would be appropriate to review the book.

Tip 2

Avoid over-quotation or paraphrasing from the actual text being reviewed. Where you do cite from the text signpost it clearly with page number(s).

Dealing with Review Editors

In most instances, Review Editors will approach you as someone already on their reviewer database/review panel or, if not, more likely as the result of being recommended by a colleague as a possible reviewer of the book. Where this is the case, it will normally be because the person approached is already an established 'expert' in the field with a known reputation for publishing. For beginning review authors (where this kind of activity forms part of their personal and professional development plans), they will most likely need to be more proactive and contact the editor directly. Most journals offer the contact details of Review Editors in their online website pages.

If you do wish to approach a Review Editor then there are a few common sense rules to follow. Firstly, ensure that you are respectful and informed.

Do not assume that your attempts to approach them will result in a 'given' opportunity to write a review. There are many factors that govern what editors can or cannot include at any given time, including, for example, where they already have a large number of reviews waiting to be published. As mentioned in Chapter 2, however, journals such as *Nurse Education in Practice* and *Journal of Clinical Nursing* have the option to publish early online versions of a review and in the case of *Nurse Education in Practice*, the reviews only get published in full in the online issue of the journal (see http://www.sciencedirect.com/science/journal/14715953/11/4 – Book Reviews (e-only); Accessed 8 November 2012).

Another very important consideration is to follow the journal book review guidelines (e.g. see Table 4.2). Guidelines may be either supplied by the

Table 4.2 Example of a Review Editor letter and guidelines.

Date:

Dear.....,

Many thanks for agreeing to review the enclosed book.

Below are the review guidelines – and I have enclosed an example of a recent review for reference.

JOURNAL OF.....................: BOOK REVIEW GUIDELINES

- The review should be 500–750 words in length and completed in 4–6 weeks.
- You can keep any book that you review. However, if you do not provide a review you may be asked to return the book.
- Please refer to recent copy of a book review in *Journal of*........... for house style.
- Please try to deal with the book's strengths and weaknesses in a balanced way.
- .... Publishing (the publisher of the *Journal of*............) gives the following advice: 'The reviewer should take care not to write anything libellous. The review should criticise the book not the author. Any criticism of the book should be backed up with an example'. Please give a page number for the example, if possible.
- At the end of the review please give your name, job title and the full name of your employer. If you are a lecturer/practitioner or hold some other form of joint appointment please give both your job titles and name both employers.
- Please email the completed review to D.Whitehead@.......... or, if this is not possible, send a hard copy and a disk copy (marked with your name and the title of the book) to:

Dean Whitehead

.... University

Many thanks again,

Dean

editor or may already be offered in the pages of a journal (hard copy or online). Guidelines are usually clear and unambiguous. As Silver (2009, p. 11) states:

> It is important to understand publishing protocols and how editors expect prospective authors to present their work for consideration.

While this might seem a fairly obvious requirement for many, it is worth stressing here. Personally, I am particularly mindful that nearly every review that has been submitted to me, I have had to edit in terms of clearly stated house-style requirements. Murray (2009) has stated that often authors do not follow the guidelines offered, which makes one consider whether they actually look at them in the first place. Writing and then formatting as requested in the guidelines may mean the difference between seeing your review in print (or online) sooner than later, which would involve the review being returned to you for re-working or checking and therefore holding up the publication process.

Table 4.3 is an anonymous example of an actual review that has complied with the house-style rules of a certain journal. Note too that it is written in a comprehensive, informative, objective and well-balanced manner. Table 4.4 is, hopefully, an obvious example of how not to submit a book review – in comparison with the previous example. Oppositely, it is written in a brief, unstructured, subjective and unbalanced manner. As an ongoing process, the other main issues to remember are timely submission as agreed in the guideline, regular communications with the Review Editor and timely checking of any returned edits or galley proofs.

Starting slow or ready to go?

This question can be answered directly once the reader has read through the earlier parts of this chapter. If you are well versed and tested in the skills of academic writing and publishing, then the likelihood is that you are 'ready to go'. That said, do be mindful of the fact that conventions and structures for media reviews do differ slightly from conventional article, editorial or short reports.

To go in blindly without taking into account the strategies stated already in this chapter would constitute a flawed and probably problematical approach to book reviewing; if not for you at least for the Review Editor. It is assumed, however, that most readers of this chapter are more at the beginning of their journey in relation to academic writing and publication. In this case, what is suggested is careful reading and note taking of the general hints and tips contained in this chapter as a useful resource for heightening the chances of successful and 'painless' submissions (see Box 4.2). Actively seeking out support will always assist further.

Table 4.3 A good example of a book review.

Book review

Edited by Dean Whitehead

Clinical Nursing Skills: A Framework for Guiding Clinical Practice by Ruth Smith, Phil Jones and Simon Brown (eds). 2012. Oxford University Press, Oxford, UK. ISBN 89777888833. 660 pp. £27.99.

Central to training to become a qualified nurse is the acquisition of a set of clinical skills and knowledge that can be used in the care of patients. The process of gaining these skills can be an intense, difficult and stressful period for the student nurse. The clinical, managerial and interpersonal skills they learn during their training have to be applied, developed and often modified in light of changing circumstances. Being able to perform a particular procedure does not necessarily mean that a student will be aware of the holistic package of care with which it may be associated. Nurses, therefore, have to be aware of what is important prior, during and after the clinical procedure. They also have to possess awareness of the associated potential problems.

This book is aimed at second and third year undergraduate nursing students as a primer for leading up to qualification and registration – and is written with the aim of providing a comprehensive description of the clinical skills necessary to care for adults in hospital and primary care. It identifies the core skills that newly qualified nurses will require based on the UK's Nursing and Midwifery Councils 'Essential Skills Clusters'. While its premise is based on the UK's clinical competencies, it aligns directly with similar requirements for professional nursing bodies internationally. The initial chapters take the reader through communication skills, the patient pathway and essential skills. The subsequent chapters are broken down into the various systems of the body. After a brief outline of the relevant anatomy and physiology, each procedure associated with a particular body system are described. The circumstances in which the related clinical skill may be needed are explained; a green tick indicates where it should be undertaken and a red cross where it should not. An icon also indicates where there may be variations in local practice and so prompts the reader to seek further clarification by referring to local guidelines and policies. In addition, a series of questions and scenarios linked to the detailed skill are provided to allow the reader to consider the theory related to clinical situations. All this is supplemented by online resources, which aim to ensure that the evidence base related to the procedures remains up-to-date. One particularly useful feature of this book is the clear, detailed step-by-step guide for the procedures. These descriptions take the form of a table in which each procedure is clearly outlined in a linear and sequential fashion – with a column providing a rationale for each of the steps. The book also includes details of the equipment that may be needed, potential communication issues, what may need doing on the completion of the procedure and a patient deterioration box highlights any warning signs.

One criticism of this book is that it sometimes switches between advanced and basic skills too quickly. It states that it is aimed at nursing students but includes information that would be more applicable to nurse specialists and those who have taken on additional, extended roles following qualification. The distinction between what would be expected of a student, newly qualified nurse and a nurse who has undergone additional training, is not always made clear. One example of this is the chapter that describes drug administration. The chapter includes a

Table 4.3 *(Continued)*

diagram and text describing that two 250 mg tablets would be needed if the dose was 500 mg. Later on a step-by-step guide is provided for administering intravenous drugs – a procedure that is an extended role and that qualified nurses can only undertake after additional training. This could potentially lead the second year student to be either confused as to what is appropriate or anxious that they may be expected to perform such procedures soon after qualification – or even prior. Although I have levelled criticism for the book being too advanced for undergraduate students in parts, the book would be a valuable resource for newly qualified nurses. Another reservation is that some of the clinical procedures described may vary between different hospitals and areas. For example the questions used in the assessment of mental capacity (AMT) are not always the same, and assessments such as phlebitis scores may be based on locally developed instruments. In summary though, this is a well-written, clear and useful clinical procedure guide that would be of use to both students and qualified staff.

Simon Pegg

Nurse Researcher/Project Manager

Clinical Research Unit

School of Health and Social Studies

University of Ireland

Ireland

Table 4.4 A poor example of a book review that would require 'heavy' editing and re-working.

Clinical Nursing Skills (Smith, Jones and Brown). Oxford

This book is a good read for those who want to know more about clinical skills. It identifies the core skills that newly qualified nurses will require based on the UK's Nursing and Midwifery Council's regulations. This would not be so good for international readers though – although might be alrigth to use in some countries outside the UK. The first chapters are useful – and better than the ones that follow. A few of them is really quite useless and could be ignored. Thos echapters, I just rushed through as they were quite boring and i didn't agree with what they were saying. The following chapters are broken down into systems after a brief outline of other factors. One thing that I particularly like is where a green tick indicates where a skill should be and a red cross where it should not. Anyone attempting the red tick skills would only have themselves to blame. I did not, however, agree with some of them and expected to see more really. There are other useful supplements – such as links to online resources – even if some of them are a bit silly.

So, overall then this the book would be a good resource for newly qualified nurses – or at least those ones that I know. I woulod be happy to recommend it. In summary, this is a well written (but not very humorous), clear and useful clinical procedure guide – so go out and order your copy today!!

Simon Pegg

Box 4.2 Writing in action

Two recent authors advocate the notion of developing academic writing skills very early on in nursing careers – starting with undergraduate nursing students. Diehl (2007) offers an anecdotal perspective of how students can improve on their academic writing skills through various practical strategies. Where nurse educators 'lament' that their students cannot write effectively, early intervention on developing academic writing skills is particularly advocated. The intention is to create, at the very least, more confident nurse writers. Griffiths and Nicholls (2010) report on their curriculum project that used up-to-date online technologies to support the academic writing of students from the university setting into their practice arena. It focused on assignment writing – but the principles could easily be applied to writing for publication at a beginning level. Bear in mind also that the reporting and the findings of these two articles can just as easily be applied to the context of postgraduate curriculum training.

Activity 4

Is this chapter written well? Be candid and honest – but be objective and balanced as well. You may also wish to consider this chapter in the wider context of the book and when it is published, choose to undertake a review for the publisher or for a journal.

Summary

Writing a media review may, at first glance or consideration, seem like a relatively straightforward exercise. The fact that this book devotes a whole chapter to the issue should go some way, however, in identifying that this is not the case – especially when done correctly. Whether writing media reviews as a fledgling author or as a veteran of publishing, it is argued here that reading this content is a worthwhile undertaking. After all 'publication is the hard currency of science' (Rhoads, 2006, p. 1). Media reviews should be seen as a useful means of learning and honing writing skills and an exercise worth doing well.

References

Baldwin, C. & Chandler, G.E. (2002) Improving faculty publication output: the role of a writing coach. *Journal of Professional Nursing*, 18(1), 8-15.

Diehl, S.H. (2007) Developing students' writing skills: an early intervention approach. *Nurse Educator*, 32, 202–206.

Driscoll, J. & Driscoll, A. (2002) Writing an article for publication: an open invitation. *Journal of Orthopaedic Nursing*, 6, 144–152.

Dunleavy, R. (2010) *Authoring a PhD. How to Plan, Draft, Write and Finish a Doctoral Thesis or Dissertation*. Basingstoke: Palgrave MacMillan.

Faigley, L. (2011) *The Little Penguin Handbook (Australasian Edition)*. Frenchs Forest: Pearson Australia.

Griffiths, L. & Nicholls, B. (2010) e-support4U: an evaluation of academic writing skills support in practice. *Nurse Education in Practice*, 10, 341–348.

Grympna, S. (2007) Publish or perish: confessions of a new academic. *Nurse Author & Editor*, 17(2), 1–3.

Hawkins, J.W. (2009) You use APA and I use AMA. *Nurse Author & Editor*, 19(4), 1–3.

Heinrich, K.T., Neese, R., Rogers, D. & Facente, A. (2004) Turn accusations into affirmations: transform nurses into published authors. *Nurse Education Perspectives*, 25, 139–145.

Heyman, B. & Cronon, P. (2005) Writing for publication: adapting academic work into articles. *British Journal of Nursing*, 14, 400–403.

Holland, K. (2010). Dissemination of evidence : writing for publication and presentation of learning activity, Chapter 10. In: Holland, K. & Rees, C. (Eds.), *Nursing: Evidence-Based Practice Skills*. Oxford: Oxford University Press, pp. 248–285.

Keen, A. (2007) Writing for publication: pressures, barriers and support strategies. *Nurse Education Today*, 27, 382–388.

McGrail, M.R., Rickard, C.M. & Jones, R. (2006) Publish or perish: a systematic review of interventions to increase academic publication rates. *Higher Education Research & Development*, 25(1), 19–35.

McVeigh, C., Moyle, K., Forrester, K., Chaboyer, W., Patterson, E. & St John, W. (2002) Publication syndicates: in support of nursing scholarship. *Journal of Continuing Education in Nursing*, 33(2), 63–66.

Miracle, V. (2003) Writing for publication. You can do it. *Dimensions of Critical Care Nursing*, 22(1), 31–34.

Murray, R. (2002) *How to Write a Thesis*. Berkshire: Open University Press.

Murray, R. (2009) *Writing for Academic Journals*, 2nd edition. Berkshire: Open University Press.

Nelms, B.C. (2004) Writing for publication: your obligation to the profession (Editorial). *Journal of Paediatric Health Care*, 18, 1–2.

Parker, V., Giles, M., Parmenter, G., Paliadelis, P. & Turner, C. (2010) (W)riting across and within: providing a vehicle for sharing locval nursing and midwifery projects and innovation. *Nurse Education in Practice* 10, 327–332.

Polit, D. & Northam, S. (2010) Publication opportunities in nonnursing journals. *Nurse Educator*, 35, 237–242.

Regan, M. & Pietrobon, R. (2010) A conceptual framework fro scientific writing in nursing. *Journal of Nursing Education*, 49, 437–443.

Rhoads, J. (2006) Scholarly publication. *Nurse Author & Editor*, 16(2), 1–4.

Robson, C. (2007) *How to do a Research Project: A Guide for Undergraduate Students*. Oxford: Blackwell Publishing Ltd.

Salamonson, Y., Koch, J., Weaver, R., Everett, B. & Jackson, D. (2009) Embedded academic writing support for nursing students with English as a second language. *Journal of Advanced Nursing*, 66, 413–421.

Savitz, D.A. (2000) Failure to publish results of epidemiological studies is unethical. *Epidemiology and Society*, 11, 361–363.

Silver, J. (2009) Secrets of successful writers. *Nurse Author & Editor*, 19(4), 9–12.

Taylor, J., Lyon, P. & Harris, J. (2004) Writing for publication: a new skill for nurses? *Nurse Education in Practice*, 5, 91–96.

Whitehead, D. (2000) Academic writing. *Professional Nurse*, 16, 849–851.

Whitehead, D. (2002) The academic writing experiences of a group of student nurses: a phenomenological study. *Journal of Advanced Nursing*, 38, 498–506.

Whitehead, D., Elliott, D. & Schneider, Z. (2007) Writing and presenting research findings for dissemination. In: Schneider, Z., Whitehead, D., Elliott, D., LoBiondo-Wood, G. & Haber, J. (Eds.) *Nursing & Midwifery Research: Methods and Appraisal for Evidence-Based Practice*, 3rd edition. Sydney: Elsevier – Mosby, pp. 374–389.

Websites

REF UK. Available at: http://www.hefce.ac.uk/research/ref/ [Accessed 9 June 2012].

PBRF – New Zealand. Available at: http://www.tec.govt.nz/Funding/Fund-finder/Performance-Based-Research-Fund-PBRF-/ [Accessed 9 June 2012].

Answers to activities

Activity 1

Personal experience/observation exercise that does not require suggested answers.

Activity 2

Personal experience/observation exercise that does not require suggested answers.

Activity 3

(1) Is the text original, topical and up-to-date? If the text is more than a year or so old (it takes about 2-years to get it into print in the first instance) – then it may already have been superseded or may be considered out-of-date. Where a topic market is 'flooded', it is often more difficult to review a text in terms of 'how different it is'. This might mean reviewing at least a proportion of these other texts to be able to compare and contrast, adding to the complexity of the overall task.

(2) Does the text reflect the nature of the journal to review it, that is, is it clinical, international, discipline-specific, etc. – or whatever the journal aims for in terms of its audience, scope and structure?

(3) Does the text interest you enough to want to read it critically and thoroughly?

(4) Is the text manageable to digest and critically review within the stated deadline time, that is, is it concise or a weighty tome?

(5) Can you make the review interesting for the reader? As Grympna (2007, p. 3) eloquently states:

> While publication itself may seem an admirable goal, aiming for publication alone is actually rather short sighted. Ideally we must aim to bring something of value to our readers.

(6) Does your target journal (or other format) publish media reviews? This might seem like a 'no-brainer' but I do know myself where individuals have sent reviews for journals that have discontinued reviews some time previously and, in some case, where journals have never published these types of reviews before. Perhaps those authors thought that their submissions might spark off a 'chain reaction'!!

(7) Can you readily access previous 'house-style' examples – and are you able to easily follow that format?

(8) Can you keep to any stated word limit?

(9) Can you meet any stated time deadline?

(10) Copyright – ensure that you have not sent this review anywhere else.

(11) Are any 'hidden' (or otherwise) costs of production to be met by you or your organisation? This is particularly the case with online-only publishing companies.

(12) Do you have clear contact details and format instructions to send copy to the Review Editor(s)?

Activity 4

Personal experience/observation exercise that does not require suggested answers.

Chapter 5

Writing for Publication: The Journal Article

Roger Watson

Faculty of Health and Social Care, University of Hull, Hull, UK

Introduction

This chapter covers the essential features of writing an original article for a journal. Original articles are not the only items that journals publish, but they are the most common, alongside reviews, discursive articles and other shorter pieces such as editorials, commentaries and brief reports. However, being the most common, the original article is the item you are most likely to contribute to a journal and the features of it underpin most of the features of writing other types of contributions.

These common features will be discussed in the context of writing an original article for publication and will follow a logical sequence (see Recommended reading list to supplement the guidance offered in this chapter). The chapter is conveniently considered in three sections: the first around publishing protocols and writing an article (things to consider before you start writing), the second around the protocols of writing the article itself and its organisation, and the third around the actual writing of the article itself.

What message and to whom?

It is important to be clear on what message you want to convey in your article and at whom you want to aim it. You may spend some time deciding on this before you write, but I would not let that detract you from writing; it is often only in getting something written that you can then look at it and revise it in line with the message and the audience. Keep this in mind throughout the process right up to the final revision.

In terms of the message, it is common that what you are trying to convey in one article may only be part of a larger study, for example a PhD or a larger

Writing for Publication in Nursing and Healthcare: Getting It Right, First Edition.
Edited by Karen Holland and Roger Watson.
© 2012 John Wiley & Sons, Ltd. Published 2012 by John Wiley & Sons, Ltd.

funded research project. You should always make it clear that what you are writing is from a larger study, and therefore, one in a series of articles and do not try to convey too much in a single article. Be clear on the aims and objectives; write them down at the start and this should help you to maintain focus.

With reference to the audience, it is important to select the right type of journal and this can be achieved by reading the aims and scope of a few relevant journals carefully. The aims and scope of *Journal of Advanced Nursing*, *Nurse Education Today* and *Gastroenterology Nursing* are shown in Box 5.1. Broadly speaking, there are generic journals (e.g. *Journal of Advanced Nursing* and *International Journal of Nursing Studies*), specialist clinical journals

---

Box 5.1 Examples of journal aims and scope

Journal of Advanced Nursing

The editors welcome papers that advance knowledge and understanding of all aspects of nursing and midwifery care, research, practice, education and management. All papers must have a sound scientific, theoretical or philosophical base.

Nurse Education Today

The journal aims to publish high-quality original research and reviews, debate and discussion in nursing, midwifery and health professional education. With an international authorship and readership, the *journal* welcomes scholarly contributions that are local, national or international in scope but are of wide interest and reflect the diversity of people, health and education systems worldwide.

The *journal* wishes to encourage research of all traditions and will publish papers that show depth, rigour, originality and high standards of presentation. In particular, the journal will publish work that is analytical and constructively critical of both previous work and current initiatives.

The editors and referees welcome works of research, policy, theory and philosophy of health professional education that meet and develop the high academic and ethical standards of the *journal*.

The *journal* also publishes reviews of learning and teaching media and books. Together with other organisations, the journal seeks to extend the boundaries of quality and availability of research and scholarship in nursing, midwifery and health professional education.

Gastroenterology Nursing

The journal keeps gastroenterology nurses and associates informed of the latest developments in research, evidence-based practice techniques, equipment, diagnostics and therapy.

(e.g. *Gastroenterology Nursing* and *International Journal of Nursing Older People*) and nursing educational journals (e.g. *Nurse Education Today*, *Journal of Nursing Education* and *Nurse Education in Practice*). Therefore, just because your article is about nursing it is not necessarily the case that any journal will consider it. Also, some journals such as the *Journal of Clinical Nursing*, despite the title, are actually quite generic in their content, with a special focus, however, on clinical practice and relevance to clinical practice articles.

Therefore, it is essential to read the aims and scope of a journal carefully and, if in any doubt, take a look at a few issues of the journal and decide if the kind of articles published are similar in format to your article, would convey your ideas and reach your target audience. In these days of online publishing and searching it is possibly not so important to go for a journal that specialises in your field, such as *Nurse Education Today* for an educational article. However, those with a specific interest in nursing education are more likely to scan the contents of educational journals more regularly.

Moreover, generic journals tend to have much greater levels of article submission; therefore, you are competing against other types of articles and in much greater numbers. Finally, there is nothing wrong with sending an abstract of your article to the journal to ask if it is suitable or contacting the editor initially to inquire whether this is the type of article they would be interested in publishing in their journal.

> ### Tip 1
>
> This kind of activity is very important in pre-writing preparation, as ensuring your article meets the aims and scope of a journal together with choosing one that reaches the most appropriate audience for your 'message' are essential first steps to successful publication.

Targeting a journal

While there is no guarantee of being published in any journal to which you submit a manuscript, it is essential that you have a specific one in mind when you are preparing your manuscript. You may have considered several of these for submission of your work, but in the process of preparation, you need to be very clear about which one you are writing for. This is logical if you consider the information available when you consult journal guidelines and how these can help you to focus your article appropriately and how specific these guidelines are to any particular journal.

If this is your first attempt at writing an article, then decide where it may be submitted. You will, inevitably, have to alter it, sometimes substantially or it may even get rejected when first submitted because you had not prepared properly. This, in fact, wastes a great deal of time, not only for you in trying to get your work published but also for the editor and reviewers (if it gets to that point), and increases chances of being rejected.

Tip 2

Decide on message to be conveyed in the article, who the audience is to read it, read aims and scope of a few possible journals, read some articles that have similar type of message you wish to convey in them, write the article to meet the specific aims and scope. This shows the editor that you have undertaken some preparation, and for first time authors, this is essential good practice.

Some people advocate starting at the most popular or prestigious journals in your field of interest first (often those that have large numbers of papers submitted because of this) and then working down the list of popularity until one of them accepts your final article. While you may be lucky with this approach, you must appreciate that the more prestigious the journal the more likely you are to be rejected. There are, of course, exceptions to this, particularly if your article is well written, may discuss a major breakthrough in scientific knowledge and/or meets the general high standards of that journal. When talking about prestigious journals, it is normally about those which have an 'impact factor' (see Chapter 2), which is those journals that have been deemed to be acceptable for including in the impact factor table. At present, there are only 89 journals in the Nursing subject list of Thomson Impact Factor journals (accessed via Athens 18 November 2011), and although this is indicative of an overall high-quality indicator, not every country in the world now uses this as the only barometer of a prestigious journal to publish your work. However, regardless of what one considers to be a prestigious journal, for many countries, publishing in these impact factor rated journals is still the goal for many aspiring new authors and, for others, essential for their future careers.

More experienced authors may be better able to judge where their work will be accepted and – being well published themselves – will not be in such a hurry to have their next article published as less experienced authors, who are developing their curriculum vitae (CV) or academic/clinical practice profiles.

Nevertheless, do not get into the habit of underselling your work by always submitting to journals where you are most likely always to be accepted because they are viewed by yourself and others as less prestigious; ultimately, this may not be to your advantage as you build you research and writing career. This applies to writing for both generic content and specialist journals.

You will suffer rejection at points in your writing for publication career, but reflecting on the 'four rules' of writing (Chapter 2), treat rejection as the start of the next submission. Therefore, if your article is rejected, and we all receive rejections, regardless of how experienced we are at writing for publication, you will need to target another journal. You may not choose to do so immediately but it is important not to allow the article you have worked hard to write linger in a desk drawer for months on end! You will, however, need to reconsider where you are going to try getting it published next, and if it has been out to review you may have received the reviewer's comments that you can consider in any future revision and re-submission elsewhere. You wrote the manuscript because you believed the contents to be of value to others, therefore, so re-visit the main messages in your paper, find a new journal, read the new guidelines and alter your manuscript appropriately.

Read the guidelines

The pattern for preparing an original article for publication described here is quite typical for any journal but if you are unsure then follow the first of the 'four rules' (Chapter 2): *read the guidelines*. The importance of reading the guidelines was explained in Chapter 2, but it is reiterated here with specific regard to the writing of an original article.

Therefore, taking the above advice, it is worth considering what visiting the guidelines page of a typical academic journal will show you and what features you should be looking for.

Section 1: Reading the guidelines

First, find the guidelines pages of the journal where you plan to submit your article, they are normally found at the back of a printed journal (not in every issue) or in many journals on the journal website (see examples at *International Journal of Nursing Studies* website: http://www.elsevier.com/wps/find/journaldescription.cws_home/266/authorinstructions and *Journal of Advanced Nursing* website: http://onlinelibrary.wiley.com/journal/10.1111/(ISSN) 1365-2648/homepage/ForAuthors.html):

(1) The first feature that you should look for is the permitted maximum word limit of articles accepted and if there are any variations to this. For example, some journals publish short reports or permit longer articles in consultation with the editor. An example of this is a systematic review, due to often large tables of critically reviewed papers and an explanation of the search process undertaken. Knowing the maximum permitted length, which you should not feel obliged to reach, provides your first aim. However, it is important that the length of the article is not too short either, as it may not convey enough detail for the reviewers to make a fair assessment of its value for publication (see Chapter 12). A useful exercise can be seen in Box 5.2 to help you with this issue.

Box 5.2   Using the aims and scope of some journals

Using these links to some popular journals see if you can find the aims and scope of:

Nurse Education in Practice: http://www.nurseeducationinpractice.com/
Journal of Clinical Nursing: http://onlinelibrary.wiley.com/journal/10.1111/
  (ISSN)1365-2702
Journal of Nursing Education: http://www.slackjournals.com/jne
Research in Nursing and Health: http://onlinelibrary.wiley.com/journal/
  10.1002/(ISSN)1098-240X

(2) The second feature from the guidelines that you need to ascertain is the organisation of the article. This was mentioned briefly in Chapter 2; the organisation under headings and sub-headings is usually provided in the guidelines but if you are in any doubt, make sure you read some articles from the journal and look at how authors have structured their writing; it should be obvious if the journal insists on one form of organisation or if there is any flexibility and differences between types of articles. The organisation of an article is very important; it gives the articles 'direction' so that the reader is oriented from start to finish and so that you can, concomitantly, organise the contents in this way. The organisation of an article under main headings is also important for the rapid retrieval of information from the article, especially the abstract that is used in online databases. The format for an abstract is considered later in the chapter.

Activity 1

Compare the word limits expected for main article submission in each journal in Box 5.2, and also for other sections of the journals, such as research reports, debate issues or commentaries. Consider how your work could be written for these different sections.

It is quite common for academic articles not to be read entirely by journal readers; instead, some people may only read the Aims and the Conclusion to come to a judgement, and some may only be interested in the Design and Methods. It depends very much on why they are accessing the journal and the article in the first place.

You should help people to find information quickly by ensuring that you write the appropriate content under the appropriate headings. However, some journals do not have specific requirements of headings, but there is still an expected protocol for construction of an article and especially the abstract.

Tip 3

Once again, if in any doubt about what parts of your proposed article go under which sections in the submitted manuscript, you are advised to read a few articles in the journal that you are aiming at and re-visit the author guidelines.

What else do journal guidelines tell us? In addition to the permitted length of a manuscript, journal guidelines should tell you all that you need to know, from the structure of the manuscript and the types of submissions they accept for publication to the minutiae of editorial requirements. Increasingly, publishers will have standard guidelines for certain aspects of manuscripts that are common to all journals that they publish and there will often be electronic links to these. Therefore, it is essential to read the journal guidelines online so that you can easily access these links while you are reading the main guidelines; see Box 5.3 for an example regarding word length from *Journal of Clinical Nursing* (a Wiley-Blackwell journal).

Box 5.3   Permitted length of manuscripts

This section comes from the online author guidelines for *Journal of Clinical Nursing* at http://onlinelibrary.wiley.com/journal/10.1111/(ISSN)1365-2702/homepage/ForAuthors.html

Please note that quotations are included in the overall word count of articles.

Original articles: These articles should be between 3000 and 5000 words long, double spaced with a wide margin (at least 2 cm) on each side of the text. The main text should be structured as follows: Introduction (putting the paper in context – policy, practice or research); Background (literature); Methods (design, data collection and analysis); Results; Discussion; Conclusion; Relevance to clinical practice. The number of words used, excluding abstract, references, tables and figures, should be specified. Pilot studies are not suitable for publication as original articles.

Review articles: Qualitative and quantitative literature reviews on any area of research relevant to clinical nursing and midwifery are welcomed. Submissions should not exceed 5000 words, excluding abstract, tables, figures and reference list. Quotes are included in the overall word count of the main text.

Box 5.4 An example of how to layout a manuscript

Introduction

The use of questionnaires is important and widespread in nursing research and practice. A well-designed questionnaire is a valuable instrument for the measurement of phenomena such as psychological morbidity, quality of life and clinical symptoms. Also, in nursing and other areas of social research, the measurement of attitudes, opinions and educational achievement is common and valuable.

The development of questionnaires requires some obligatory steps including the clarification of the concept being studied, the selection of items, validation of content, establishing the reliability of the items, and then further steps to investigate the construct validity of the questionnaire. This field of research is known as psychometrics and depends heavily on methods developed in psychology that are equally applicable across the different fields where questionnaires are used. The methods employed to ensure that questionnaires are psychometrically sound range from common sense (selection of items and validation of content) to some sophisticated mathematical and statistical methods for establishing reliability and validity.

Classical test theory

The methods used to establish reliability and validity rely heavily on what is referred to as classical test theory, which includes methods such as Cronbach's alpha for the estimation of reliability of a test score. Classical test theory – which will not be expounded on further here – is concerned with the estimation of measurement error and establishing, within the bounds of the methods available, an estimate of the true score.

The guidelines will advise on the preferred layout for manuscripts. Even with online and electronic submissions, it is common for double spacing to be required with wide margins to the text, as shown in Box 5.4. Also, a font size and type will be specified. You should get these superficial aspects of your submission right. Presenting your manuscript in the correct format impresses the editorial staff that you have read the guidelines and that you have paid them the compliment of following them.

Editorial staff are busy, often dealing with thousands of manuscripts annually – hundreds weekly – and do not have the time to do this for you. If your manuscript does not look like a submission to the journal it will – and quite fairly – be returned to you for amendment, if you are lucky; if you are unlucky it will be rejected even before it goes out to a reviewer. The editorial process and decisions will be covered in Chapter 10.

The next major aspect of a manuscript is the organisation under headings and sub-headings and this will be covered in Section 2 (Writing and organising the article). However, beyond these aspects of the manuscript lie layers of editors' and publishers' preferences and requirements that you need to pay attention to and only some of these can be covered here. First, you may need to pay attention to spelling – does the journal adopt US or UK English (see http://www.blackwellpublishing.com/pdf/house_style_uk.pdf and http://authorservices.wiley.com/bauthor/House_style_guide_ROW45201014 51415.pdf; Accessed 23 April 2012)? This is, largely, a function of the country where the editorial office is located and if the office is in the United States they are usually not as tolerant of UK spelling. The main differences lie in the use of specific word spellings for same sounding name (dipthongs), for example 'color' for 'colour'; and the use if 'z' in endings as in 'recognize' as opposed to 'recognise'. It is unfortunate that many grammar and spelling check systems on computers use one form only.

Section 2: Writing and organising the article

Organising a manuscript

Organising a manuscript was briefly mentioned with respect to getting started with writing for publication (Chapter 2) and how useful setting out a basic framework for a manuscript was, using the guidelines for organisation given by a journal. Now I will look at what should be included under the various sections of a manuscript and use the headings as shown in Box 5.5.

Box 5.5   The organisation of contents of a typical paper

Title
Abstract
Introduction*
Background*
The Study*
Results*
Discussion*
Conclusion*
Acknowledgement
Contributions
References
Figures and Tables

In Box 5.1, the asterisked sections are those that usually contribute to the word count but this specific point is worth checking with the journal guidelines or if not published specifically, with the editorial office. Some journals do include all aspects of the manuscript in the word count and some journals specify a page extent as opposed to a word count. This is an important issue to consider pre-writing stage, given word writing plans as discussed in Chapter 2.

Another general point to note is that tables and figures are not normally integrated throughout the manuscript; they are usually presented at the end following the references – but this can also differ between journals.

Tip 4

The message again to reiterate is: the first of the 'four rules': read the guidelines. Box 5.6 provides a checklist of the various aspects to be described next; these are key points about the actual writing of the article specifically.

The title

Titles are important: they should be as short and informative as possible (Watson, 2010). You want potential readers to find your article, to read and understand the title and then to read and possibly cite your article. The title helps you to achieve all of this. Therefore, think carefully about your title and revise it prior to submission. Reviewers may recommend title changes, especially if they consider that the content of the article they have reviewed does not reflect the title itself.

Sometime editors, either acting on reviewers comments or on their own judgement, will suggest that you alter your title or, if minor, will do this for you but if this is substantial then they should consult you. In doing this, the editor is attempting to improve the title, make it fit the style of the journal and increase the 'discoverability' (see Section 'Discoverability') of your article.

It is becoming increasingly common for the important aspect of the article to appear first in the title, that is at the left-hand side, so that this is read first and this also ensures that it appears on a web page and is not obscured or runs off the page. Remember, all searching for articles is now undertaken via the Internet or organisational databases from publishers and you should take this into account when writing your article, if you want it read by the international community. For example, if your article is a literature or systematic review or a randomised controlled trial then these are the important aspects of the article that you want to convey. People finding your article will already be searching for the subject material and will be drawn towards both reviews and randomised controlled trials. For example, rather than *Non-pharmacological treatment for depression: a systematic review*, it is better to use *A systematic review of non-pharmacological treatment for depression*. Likewise, rather than writing *Paracetamol versus aspirin: a randomised*

Box 5.6 Example of checklist for preparing a typical manuscript

Title	Is the title short and descriptive of the contents of the manuscript with the vital information at the start?
Abstract	Is this organised properly (under headings if the journal requires it) and including, at a minimum, Aims, Design, Methods, Results and Conclusion?
Introduction	Does this set the paper in its widest context, for example policy, practice, research or education?
Background	Is the relevant and only the relevant literature included here and does it end with your research question?
The Study	Is the design clearly stated and are the methods described such that a reader could repeat your study?
Results	Are all the relevant results included and have you avoided discussing them here?
Discussion	Does this reiterate the aims of the study and does it discuss the findings to this study in the light of other, relevant, work? Are limitations included? Is the gap filled by the paper made clear and have you stated the implications related to the policy, practice, research or education you outlined in the Introduction?
Conclusion	Is this succinct and does it convey clearly the main messages (around three is best) of your study?
Acknowledgement	Is anyone not included as an author but who made contribution to the study mentioned appropriately here? If the study was funded, are the funders mentioned?
Contributions	Is everyone – and only those people – who contributed to the study appropriately listed here?
References	Are they all present, correct and up to date?
Figures and Tables	Have these all been referred to in the manuscript?

controlled trial it is better to use *A randomised controlled trial of paracetamol versus aspirin.*

It is unwise to attempt humour or to make literary or cultural references unless these really reflect the content of the article and you really know what you are doing with these. One excellent example is Darbyshire's use of 'Rage against the machine' in the title of an article about the problems and pitfalls of introducing nursing IT systems in Australia (Darbyshire, 2004). Rage against the machine is a North American punk-rock band and any search for their website will also find Darbyshire's article (http://www.ncbi .nlm.nih.gov/pubmed/14687289; Accessed 23 April 2012). There are few examples of this kind of title and it is safer to adhere to short informative titles whenever possible. Of course, as in all things, some longer titles can still convey the message of the content of the article itself.

Activity 2

Consider the following titles from a selection of journals and see if you are able to determine the actual focus and/or content of the article itself. Once you have written down the answer check out your response by reading the paper and determining whether your assessment was correct or not.

(1) Comparison of post-dural puncture headache and low back pain between 23 and 25 gauge Quincke spinal needles in patients over 60 years: Randomized, double-blind controlled trial *International Journal of Nursing Studies*, Volume 48, Issue 11, Pages 1315-1322, November 2011.

(2) Manias E, Botti M & Bucknall (2002) Observation of pain assessment and management – the complexities of clinical practice. *Journal of Clinical Nursing*, 11, 724-733.

(3) Banning M (2003) Pharmacology education: a theoretical framework of applied pharmacology and therapeutics. *Nurse Education Today*, 23, 459-466.

Abstract

The abstract should, like the title, be as short and as informative as possible (Watson, 2006). Normally, the journal will specify a length for abstracts and this may be very short, say 100 words, or more generous, up to 300 words. Currently, it is very unlikely to be more than this as, if possible, the abstract should easily fit one printed page and also one page on the Internet. For examples, *Research in Nursing & Health* requests an abstract (unstructured) of 120 words and *Journal of Clinical Nursing* requests an abstract (structured) of 300 words. A clear focused abstract whether structured with headings already directed or not but has the same key issues reported, is absolutely essential, as most of the major databases are searched through their abstracts that enable researchers and authors to determine whether that article is relevant or not to their work. From there they can then access the full-text article, which because of this clarity of the abstract will not be wasted time nor resource.

Increasingly, journals require abstracts to be structured (see Box 5.7) and if they do not request a structure, then it is advisable to have a structure in

Box 5.7 Examples of structured abstracts

Journal of Clinical Nursing[a]

Aim: This article presents the findings of a systematic review of the literature on suicidal behaviour in old age, specifically examining gender differences.

Background: Numerous studies have reported that older people are at a higher risk for suicide than other age groups in most countries. Rarely do they examine whether there are differences in suicidal behaviour among older males and females.

Design: Systematic review.

Methods: Electronic databases were systematically searched to identify English language reports of research about suicide and suicide attempts in old age. Studies were assessed for inclusion on the basis of inclusion criteria. Key results concerning suicide in old age were extracted and synthesised.

Results: Twenty-two gender-specific studies on suicidal behaviour in old age were identified. All studies were of the quantitative type. Five factors affecting suicide by gender in old age were identified from the selected papers.

Conclusions: Most findings concluded that older males had a higher risk of suicide than older females. Some findings nevertheless revealed that the risk factors for one socio-demographic group may be less relevant to others and that people operate differently in different social contexts. Further in-depth exploration on the gender-specific characteristics in old-age suicide is recommended.

Relevance to clinical practice: Health professionals are encouraged to increase their knowledge of the risk factors leading to suicide in old age in their local contexts and to be able to identify potential victims and render timely and appropriate intervention. They should also be ready to open up their service boundaries and develop collaborative partnerships with local agencies and the general public.

International Journal of Nursing Studies[b]

Background

Developing a therapeutic relationship with consumers is considered as the central aspect of nursing work in mental health. The importance of this relationship stems from its association with enhanced patient care and improved patient outcomes. Factors within the practice environment may influence the nurse's ability to engage effectively in this relationship.

(*continued*)

Objective

This study explored a model that added characteristics of the individual and practice environment to a central framework incorporating therapeutic commitment: a nurse's ability and willingness to engage in a therapeutic relationship.

Setting and participants

Data were collected at six mental health nursing units in five public general acute hospitals in New South Wales, Australia, for 14 days per unit between 2005 and 2006. All nurses in participating wards were invited to partake in the study. Seventy-six (51%) responses were analysed.

Method

The data were collected using a *Nurse Survey* inclusive of the Practice Environment Scale of the Nursing Work Index, and the Mental Health Problems Perception Questionnaire. A *Unit Profile* form was used concurrently to collect staffing, skill mix and patient turnover data. Partial least squares path modelling (PLS-PM) was chosen as the analytical method to test the model and identify the most influential factors.

Results

Experienced nurses who perceived themselves to be competent and supported were more likely to express a willingness to engage therapeutically with patients. Environmental factors associated with these perceptions included foundations of quality nursing care, opportunities to participate in hospital affairs and clinical supervision. Not all elements in the proposed model were supported.

Conclusion

Positive hospital practice environments can improve the capacity of nurses working in mental health to engage therapeutically with patients. Specific approaches may include access to preceptorship, continued education and career development opportunities, together with clinical supervision, improved continuity of care and the involvement of mental health nurses in the governance of the hospital.

[a]Fung, Y.-L. & Chan, Z.C.Y. (2011) A systematic review of suicidal behaviour in old age: a gender perspective. *Journal of Clinical Nursing.* doi: 10.1111/j.1365-2702.2010.03649.x.

[b]Roche, M., Duffield, C. & White, E. (2011) Factors in the practice environment of nurses working in inpatient mental health: A partial least squares path modeling approach. *International Journal of Nursing Studies.* doi: 10.1016/j.ijnurstu.2011.07.001.

mind and to follow that. At the top of most abstracts, the first heading will be the 'purpose', 'aims' or 'objectives' of the study or the review or theoretical concepts depending on the type of paper that is being written. This is to make the aim of the study/article content obvious and applies to the printed page but especially to the Internet as noted above in relation to the major databases but also to major search engines such a Google Scholar.

It is important to bear in mind that the first reader of your article, in the form of a manuscript (submitted electronically on the majority of major journals, where often the abstract is submitted as an independent file), will be an editor followed by a reviewer and if neither of these is clear about the aim of the manuscript then it is likely to be rejected. Therefore, the abstract has an additional value of being the first stage to determining whether or not the full article meets the overall aims and scope of the journal (see Chapter 12).

Likewise, if a specified structure for your abstract is not followed then the editor who receives the article (and on some large journals there are more than one editor) is likely to reject the manuscript without being sent out to review at all; if you have not been able to follow the instructions for the abstract then you are unlikely to have followed the remaining guidelines for the manuscript. You have this one opportunity, for your article submission, to make a first impression and you need to make that first impression a positive one.

The other sub-headings are, likewise, important and some journals also ask for separate statements regarding the 'design' and the 'methods'. It is essential to make a clear statement about the design, and in common with other aspects to the preliminaries to articles, this should be as short and informative as possible; for example randomised controlled trial; systematic review; longitudinal panel survey, grounded theory, ethnography.

Methods should, likewise, be briefly and clearly stated, for example questionnaires, telephone interviews, focus groups or participant observation, and the analysis should be stated, for example descriptive, correlational, multivariate or narrative analysis or thematic content analysis. 'Results' is a common sub-heading for the abstract and here the main results should just be stated and there will usually be a conclusion section where the main implications of the study can be stated. Therefore, it could be said that the abstract is a short replica of the whole of the article and that regardless of whether structured or unstructured both should reflect the overall content.

Tip 5

It is wise to have a working abstract when you begin writing your manuscript and this can help to remind you what the main points are under the sections of the main manuscript. You must re-check the abstract before submission both to check that it accurately reflects the contents to the manuscript and to make it as clear and concise as possible.

Discoverability

Before moving on to the main body of the manuscript it is useful to consider the discoverability of the article once it is published (http://tiny.cc/fimce; Accessed 14 May 2011). In the process of submission, you will be asked to provide key words and these serve two purposes: they help the editor to find appropriate reviewers and they also help people to find your article when they search for it - which will, inevitably, be via the Internet and major databases.

Usually, a specific number of key words will be requested and you must ensure that the key words reflect the content of the article. Some journals will specify MeSH (Medical Subject Headings) for key words, and it is wise to use these where possible, as this will ensure that the article is found on commercial medical and health databases such as PubMed and CINAHL. However, it is also possible to use non-MeSH terms if these will make your article more discoverable by other search engines. Most researchers would admit to making search engines such as Google® or Google Scholar® their 'first port of call' (their initial starting point) when trying to locate articles, and this will often be done using a single search term. If there is such a search term that is relevant to your article and you have not used it, then your article will be harder to find.

Given the widespread and common use of search engines, there are other things you must ensure to make your article as discoverable as possible on the Internet and these include paying attention to the words in the title and those in the abstract.

Tip 6

To increase discoverability, it is advised that you focus on two – to three key words and to ensure that these are used - and repeated if possible - in the title, the abstract and the key words. Therefore, ensure that, certainly within the parameters of the title, abstract and key words, that you are consistent and do not change your terminology. For example, if the title of your article refers to 'older people' then ensure that this is used to describe this group in the abstract and the key words; do not vary the terminology, for example, by saying 'older adults' and 'the elderly' elsewhere. It is good practice to be consistent in your terminology throughout the manuscript too. However, you must not be gratuitous in the use of these terms; the title and the abstract need to make sense, as does the main body of the manuscript. Boxes 5.8 and 5.9 provide examples of a poorly optimised and a well-optimised abstract, respectively.

Introduction and background

It is not uncommon for some articles to only have an introduction and some a background. However, some journals require both and these do serve different purposes.

Box 5.8 Poorly optimised abstract (adapted from http://blackwellpublishing.com:443/bauthor/seo.asp)

Title: False remembering in the *senior population*

Researchers studying human memory have increasingly focused on its accuracy in *senior populations*. In this article, we briefly review the literature on such accuracy in healthy older adults. The prevailing evidence indicates that, compared with younger adults, older adults exhibit both diminished accuracy and greater susceptibility to misinformation. In addition, older adults demonstrate high levels of confidence in their false memories. We suggest an explanatory framework for the high levels observed in older adults, a framework based on the theory that consciously controlled uses of memory decline in later life, making older adults more susceptible to false memories that rely on automatic processes. We also point to future research that may remedy such deficits in accuracy.

Key words: *ageing, recall, psychology, gerontology*

Introduction

The Introduction should set the article in its broadest context. For nursing articles, this can be any and/or all of research, practice, policy and education. The Introduction should not be too long and should not contain too many

Box 5.9 Well-optimised abstract (adapted from: http://blackwellpublishing.com:443/bauthor/seo.asp)

Title: False *memory* in *older adults*

Researchers studying human *memory* have increasingly focused on *memory* accuracy in *older* populations. In this article, we briefly review the literature on *memory* accuracy in healthy older adults. The prevailing evidence indicates that, compared with younger adults, *older adults* exhibit both diminished *memory* accuracy and greater susceptibility to misinformation. In addition, older adults demonstrate high levels of confidence in their false *memories*. We suggest an explanatory framework for the high level of *false memories* observed in *older adults*, a framework based on the theory that consciously controlled uses of *memory* decline in *older adults*, making older adults more susceptible to *false memories* that rely on automatic processes. We also point to future research that may remedy such deficits in accuracy.

Key words: *memory, false memory, older adults*. . .

references. For example, if your article addressed some aspect of policy, it is probably sufficient to cite the latest policy document about the policy that is being investigated and a brief description of its implications and a brief explanation of why this is being investigated. You may want to state a very broad aim here for the article but leave the research questions until later. The aim of the article may be congruent with the aim of the study from which the article is derived, if the study is small. However, some studies take place over several years and have multiple aims and objectives; therefore, you should ensure that the aim of the article is specific to what is being addressed in the article and not simply a restatement of the aims of the larger study.

Many authors confuse the aim of the study that they may be reporting with what they wish to discuss in their article, that is, the actual aim of the article itself. This is important for the reviewers, to be able to identify immediately the purpose of the article in order to determine whether the author has actually done this (see Chapter 12).

Some journals may not require an Introduction section, as such, but it is a good idea to structure the first section of an article such that is has a few introductory paragraphs before you involve your reader in the details of the study. The introduction serves to orient the reader (including editors and reviewers) to the main purpose of the article and helps them to make sense of the details.

Background

The Background is the literature review or broad overview of general literature pertaining to the topic being written about, and which forms the basis for the article. The Background should pick up on what you have said in the Introduction and expands on it. For example, if you set your article in a policy context, the Background is the place to provide the history to the policy and to describe any relevant research in that area of policy. The literature does not have to be reviewed systematically for the background to an article, but there are times when it might be appropriate to describe a search strategy. For example, if literature is very hard to find in an area or you wish to establish the level of evidence regarding claims made about an area, then some degree of systematic searching may be appropriate.

If the article is an original article, the Background is the place to consider the research already carried out in the area you are investigating, what is known and what gaps need to be filled - emphasising the ones you propose to fill. This is also the place to mention the kinds of methods used to investigate the area to date - what the advantages of these methods are and what the disadvantages are. For example, if an area has only been investigated using Randomised Control Trials (RCTs), then you may wish to emphasise the limitations of this and express the need for more research on the patient experience.

Finally, unless stated otherwise in the journal guidelines, the Background should end with a clear statement of what you set out to do in your study and this is best expressed as a research question. There are other ways of

Box 5.10 Aims, objectives and research questions (fictional example)

Aim: The aim of this study was to survey nursing students about their experience of the new curriculum in nursing.

Objectives: The objectives of the study were to design and validate a questionnaire on student experience of the new curriculum; to distribute the questionnaire to a sample of 500 nursing students and; to correlate experience of the new curriculum with demographic data on the nursing students.

Research question: what is nursing students' experience of the new nursing curriculum?

expressing what the study is about, for example, aims and objectives or simply a statement of what the study set out to investigate. However, getting into the habit of stating a research question at the end of the Background is good practice as it makes sense of what you have been writing in the Background. Your Background should have been written to lead up to your research question – it clarifies what you are asking in your research and it helps you to set up hypotheses, for example, in quantitative research and to reflect back, from your Discussion, on the answers to the research question. The research question could be described as the pivotal point of an original article. Likewise, it is very good practice to state a research question in a literature review; it serves the same purpose as in the original article. For the distinction between aims, objectives and research a research question, see Box 5.10.

Tip 7

Remember there is a distinction between stating the aim or purpose of what you wish to discuss or present in your article from stating the aim or purpose of any research study you have undertaken. This will also apply to any theoretical or policy focused article that you have submitted.

The study

Different journals will have different conventions at this point in the article, many requesting a Methods section. Whatever the conventions of a particular journal, The Study section of an article is where the design of the research should be re-stated (from the abstract) and then the methods described in more detail than in the abstract. This is a very important part of the article and it is often read in isolation by other researchers wishing to use your method but with no specific interest in the results.

Therefore, the methods need to be described in such a way that someone reading the article could either repeat your study using this or simply use the method in their study. This applies generally to qualitative and quantitative research. Do not try to hide anything here; if something about the methods needs stating, then state it; make no assumptions, and this is especially the case if your methods are novel. Where a method is unusual or new then it may also be necessary to provide some background and this may require some theory and reference to literature that is available, maybe from another discipline.

If the method is very common – for example, a t-test is a very common statistical analysis – then there is no need to describe how to do one. Also, if the reviewers and editors are happy, then it may be possible – for some methods – to refer to other work where they are well described or to previous publications of your own where you have described them. You must be aware that reviewers spend a lot of time studying the methods sections of manuscripts to ensure that they can understand how the research has been conducted and also to see if the methods are appropriate and correctly described. Publishing research that is not considered safe in terms of the methods is not acceptable, as readers of the article are reliant on this evidence to be valid in terms of the data that then ensue from its use in the field. This is particularly important when the method may have been misunderstood by the author and their justification for it is weak.

The research design (the whole of the methodology and methods combined, along with the ethical processes etc.) is relatively simple to state, but, for example, if the study is experimental then it needs to be clear here if it is randomised, blinded, pragmatic and so on. The purpose of this is to let the reader know the extent to which the results can be generalised as well as being able to follow the method. If the study is a survey then the key aspects to emphasise are whether it is cross-sectional or longitudinal and, if longitudinal, then is the sample a trend, cohort or panel so that people will then know how much confidence they can have in the results over time.

It is essential that you are clear about your design; make the design clear and be aware of the limitations of your data – something that can then be followed through in the Discussion section. Naturally, the same applies to qualitative research; the design must be clearly stated: phenomenological, ethnographic, grounded theory. However, with regard to qualitative research there is an increasing trend among reviewers to ask authors to be very clear about the processes they went through in recording, transcribing and analysing data. In addition, it is expected that if the focus of the article has been on the findings and recommendations then the outcome of these and some evidence of how they arrived at the findings must be made clear to the reader who may also wish to use the methodology and methods used. Quantitative designs lend themselves to description by labels as there is a very common language and the designs are fixed, but people use qualitative methods very differently and this influences the analysis and interpretation of results.

Tip 8

State clearly what you have done; the analytical methods have to be described in sufficient detail for them to be understood and scrutinised by an expert. With quantitative studies, the experts often include a statistician. These points apply to both large-scale studies and smaller evaluation type studies. Regardless of size, it is good practice for any researcher to ensure that reporting of their work is accurate and that it is evident that they both understand what they have undertaken that, in turn, offers confidence to the reviewers and editor that the evidence produced and that they wish to publish is safe to do so.

Ethics

It is obligatory in most journals to describe how ethical approval was obtained for your study, if the study involved human participants (Long and Fallon, 2007). Few nursing journals will publish studies involving animals. Therefore, the body to which an ethics application was submitted and the fact that it was approved needs to be reported and if there are any unusual ethical aspects of your study then it is worth highlighting these. For example, studies involving children or vulnerable adults may have had to undergo special scrutiny and there may have been suggestions by an ethics committee of what aspects needed to be given particular attention.

It is appreciated by editors that the level of scrutiny of research projects and the precise procedures differ between countries. Therefore, journals do not prescribe the particular procedures that any study must undergo, but they do require the knowledge that the study was scrutinised by an appropriate body and that participants were protected. This applies also to non-clinical participants, such as student nurses and midwives, where University Research Committees (referred to in many countries as Institutional Review Boards) may be involved in the ethical proposal scrutiny. Without this assurance – or a credible explanation of why ethical permission was not sought (which would be unusual) – or, for example, why informed consent was not obtained (e.g. in some observational studies) then the study is unlikely to be published.

The level of evidence required by journals varies; most take the word of the author that ethical procedures have been followed, as reported in their article; after all, while publishers take their responsibility to publish ethically sound studies seriously, it is the author who will be in trouble if the procedures are not followed or if they have lied about this aspect of their study. Nevertheless, there is a trend towards being very specific about the ethics committees that were approached for permission or the processes adopted to ensure ethical good practice was conducted in the study; thereby, anyone with an interest or any doubts can actually check the veracity of the author's claim. Some journals require specific evidence, for example, the letter of permission from the ethics committee or in some journals the actual number of the ethical approval Committee.

> **Tip 9**
>
> You should retain any pieces of evidence regarding the ethical procedures related to your study, just in case you are required to provide the evidence later.

Results

The results section of a quantitative article needs to be short and to the point. Simply state your results, do not engage in any discussion. Make sure that all relevant results are reported – that is all those that will be referred to in the discussion, and no more than those. Tabulate the results as much as possible and use figures too. Ensure that all figures and tables are referred to in the results section and try only to highlight the main results from these, do not repeat everything that is tabulated in the test.

In qualitative articles, make sure that you select a few succinct quotes that convey the theme you are describing; very long quotes and multiple quotes are unnecessary, they make reading the article difficult and they occupy valuable space. Often in journals you may find the headings for a qualitative article may well be findings rather than results, and some journals have both as an either/or preferred headings.

> **Activity 3**
>
> Undertake a search using key words for methodologies and methods of your choice in both the major paradigms and qualitative and quantitative research. Identify one article of each and consider how the data have been reported.

Discussion

A good image to hold in your mind regarding the Discussion is that you are 'closing the circle'; the discussion should take the reader back to the purpose of the article and explain how that purpose has been achieved and what the significance of the results is. The discussion should be congruent with the rest of the article; avoid the mistake of introducing new ideas or new literature here; the discussion should be relevant to the research question in the light of the results of the study.

However, you may find in some articles, depending on how the author has structured it or justified their rationale for how they report the literature (as for example in the reporting of some phenomenological studies), that the editor has agreed to their use of new literature emerging in the discussion. However, it is not the normal convention for most articles.

The discussion is normally the most substantial section of the article, reminding the reader what the purpose of the article is by paraphrasing the aims or the research question at the beginning. This is a good idea as some readers may only read the discussion but it also serves to contextualise the points you wish to make in the Discussion. Following that, it is worth re-stating the main findings; again, this brings the point of the study and its main outcomes together before you discuss them.

Tip 10

Avoid repeating the results elsewhere in the discussion but make reference to them and build a story around them to convince the reader that the purpose of the study has been achieved. One trick to bear in mind, when writing the discussion, is that the purpose of the study has been achieved – whatever the outcome. In other words, if your study was an RCT and there was no difference between the treatment and control group then that is, clearly, an outcome and the purpose of the study has been achieved. Presumably your research question has been answered even if the question was does X work better than Y? If X works no better then the answer is 'no' but that is what you should report. Moreover, while you may have some difficulty publishing studies with negative results, it is still good practice to report them to avoid the 'bottom drawer' phenomenon whereby only studies that produce positive results are reported and those that do not are, metaphorically, consigned to the bottom drawer. This leads to publication bias in systematic reviews (http://www.cochrane-net.org/openlearning/html/mod15-2.htm; Accessed 23 April 2012).

You will have reviewed the literature in the Background to the study; therefore, avoid re-reviewing it in the Discussion. Instead, make reference to the main articles that either supported or refuted your reasons for conducting the study and state the extent to which your study supports prevailing views, whether it 'tips the balance' in favour of one view and what, exactly, it adds to the field of study. Be clear about making such statements but avoid overstating the results or the contribution to the field of study. This is no place for modesty but that does not mean that you should exaggerate.

It is good practice to state any limitations of the study and this, as in other sections of your discussion, can be explained under a separate sub-heading. All studies have limitations and you should be aware of that; on the other hand, do not undermine your study. The limitations are important in their own right but they also allow you to state what could be done better in future; they give you or other investigators 'threads' to pick up, whereby the study can be improved and a further contribution to the field made.

Conclusion

Most journals request a conclusion but, if not, then you should include one as good practice; if not as a separate heading then as a sub-heading at the end of the Discussion. Please note that the Conclusion is not a summary – that is the purpose of the abstract. The conclusion is the place to highlight the main findings and their relevance. If you have not already made some recommendations in the Discussion then this is the place to do that, and these can include recommendations for policy, practice, education or further research. Avoid introducing new ideas here – do not start writing another article; conclude the one you are writing – and there is no need to include any references here. Remember that many people will only read the Abstract and the Conclusions to your article; therefore, you must ensure that you make any points that you would want people to take away from your article here. This is where you demonstrate to any reader what has arisen from your study or the literature review or assessment of the theoretical evidence on which you based the premise of the content of your article. Example of conclusions from published papers are shown in Box 5.11.

Section 3: Writing the paper

Where to start

Despite the obvious order of contents of an article, it is not advisable to write the manuscript in the order of the contents. In fact, it is very helpful not to do this, which is a good tip for getting started. However, every author will eventually find their own method of writing articles or other written outputs, as we can see in this book. However, there are some basic principles in this section that will be useful for those starting out on this journey to publication.

A good place to start is with the study: the Design and Methods, as these will not change and will have been agreed before you start collecting data. Therefore, it is a good idea to write this first as you will be on 'familiar territory'; moreover, you will then have started writing your manuscript and this will make it easier to continue. Once the study section is completed you should write up the Results or findings section and this will form the basis of the remainder of the manuscript.

The order of writing the remaining contents is a matter of preference, but you could, logically, work on the Background next as, once you have written the results, you will know what literature you need to support the manuscript. Next, the Discussion can be written and then the Conclusions and Introduction. Finally, while you may have had a working abstract, you must re-visit this and ensure that it has all the essential features described earlier and also check the title and ensure that it really does reflect the contents of the manuscript.

Box 5.11 Examples of conclusions to papers

Nurse Education Today[a]

Conclusion

The overall result showed that participating lecturers judged their international exchange to be a positive experience that resulted in personal as well as professional development and form a base for future development. However, since the L-P projects are limited in time there is a risk that they might 'fade out' when their financial support ends. On the other hand, this could be a trigger for seeking and disseminating future international collaboration. A positive outcome requires an open-minded approach by participating lecturers as well as support from the organisations involved.

Nurse Education in Practice[b]

Conclusion

The SCE role can be powerful in their assistance to staff when RNs do not have particular skills. It is evident that the use of a SCE can add value to the clinical setting in addressing education needs, thereby maximising learning opportunities for students during practicum experiences. Employment of a SCE helps students' make sense of practice in clinical contexts. Further exploration around how to improve the working relationship between the RN and student is still needed, as it is the RN who is in the most significant position to enhance student learning experiences and ensure the sustainability of positive clinical practicum experiences.

[a]Enskär, K., Johansson, I., Ljusegren, G. & Widäng, I. (2011) Lecturers' experiences of participating in an international exchange. *Nurse Education Today*. doi: 10.1016/j.nedt.2010.10.018.
[b]Henderson, A. & Tyler, S. (2011) Facilitating learning in clinical practice: evaluation of a trial of a supervisor of clinical education role. *Nurse Education in Practice*. doi: 10.1016/j.nepr.2011.01.003.

Distribution of contents

There are usually no rules about how much you should write in any section of a manuscript. The abstract length and the overall length of the manuscript will be specified in the author guidelines, and you need to know whether or not the length of the manuscript includes the abstract and the reference list. My advice here assumes that the maximum permitted length of the manuscript is 5000 words (*Journal of Advanced Nursing* article word limit:

Box 5.12 Typical distribution of contents in an original paper

Introduction	500 words
Background	1000 words
Methods	500 words
Results	500 words
Discussion	2000 words
Conclusion	500 words

http://onlinelibrary.wiley.com/journal/10.1111/(ISSN)1365-2648/homepage/jan _essentials.htm; Accessed 23 April 2012) excluding the abstract and the reference list – this is quite common. Others such as *Nurse Education in Practice* have up to 4000 words including references (http://www.elsevier.com/wps/find/journaldescription.cws_home/623062/authorinstructions) but excluding abstract while the journal *Sociology of Health & Illness* accepts articles of 8000 words in length, including notes and bibliography (http://www.blackwellpublishing.com/shil_enhanced/submit.asp).

The most substantial parts of a manuscript are usually the Background and the Discussion. I find it helpful to think (and write) in 500 word units and to base the length of each section on this. This is not a 'rule' as such as, once the manuscript is written, some adjustment may be necessary and, of course, 5000 words is the maximum permitted length; you do not have to attain that, shorter manuscripts are perfectly acceptable, as long as they convey the essential content. An example of a possible distribution of contents could be as that shown in Box 5.12.

Some adjustment may be necessary but you must bear in mind that an expansion of any single section will require some reduction in words elsewhere. Similarly, if your manuscript is returned by the journal requiring amendments and these involve expanding a section then you will still have to trim elsewhere; the permitted length does not change and editors will rarely allow you to write over the word limit (see Chapter 10).

Tables and figures

Sometimes, journals will specify the number of tables and figures and other ways of summarising results that are permitted. They do this not only for the sake of clarity of reading an article but also because each issue of the journal over a period of 12 months of a volume (i.e. a number of issues per year) is only allowed a certain number of pages for publishing articles. If they allowed every author to include as many tables as they wished then the pages would be filled very quickly, reducing the number of possible articles that can be published in each issue.

Tip 11

If in doubt about the number of tables or figures it may be useful to contact the editorial office for additional advice. This would also apply to those articles in some journals where photographs of illustrations form part of the content.

Where they do not specify, then the best advice is to have enough to help readers understand the results; it is very hard to grasp a lot of quantitative data written in the results section; much better to tabulate or present in a figure. However, it is not helpful to have too many tables or figures as this can detract from reading the article. The best advice is, without over-complicating the presentation, to try to get as much information into as few tables as possible. Therefore, whenever possible, gather all congruent data in a single table and a good example of this are the demographic data. It is not helpful to distribute this over several tables; therefore, find ways of indicating the gender distribution of participants and also to indicate the separate features of the men and the women in one table, for example.

In longitudinal studies, avoid presenting the waves separately; find some way of gathering all the data for one aspect of the study in a single table. Be meticulous about the numbers in the columns - make sure they add up and if, for example, numbers are less than or greater than 100% of the number of participants, check this and if this is really the case - for example where individuals may have more than one diagnosis then provide an explanation for this.

There are some rules about tables and figures: do not repeat too much of what is tabulated in the text - just emphasise the main points; do not use a figure and a table to present the same data; and refer to all figures and tables in your manuscript. In addition, use tables and figures to good effect - there is no preference for one over the other; whichever is best and this may require some experimenting and possibly advice.

In figures, use monochrome unless absolutely necessary; colour is expensive to produce and does not preserve well in hard copy. Some journals may actually charge you for including colour diagrams or photographs, but the advent of new technology does mean that more and more journals can use colour in various ways on their electronic version of the articles.

Keep figures simple - three-dimensional bar charts may look impressive in glossy magazines and power point presentations, but they are unnecessary in an academic article. For qualitative research findings, it is normally the narratives of participants that are presented and a balance must be made between using a large amount of quotations that are used to illustrate themes arising from the data for discussion and what are absolutely vital ones to illustrate a specific finding. Experience in writing over time will enable authors to identify one or two quotes from many, which capture meaning of the findings very well.

Activity 4

Access the journals noted in Box 5.2 and find articles that have used both tables and figures and others that have used participant narratives or quotations. Look at how much space they take up in the article and also most importantly what they contribute to the findings.

The reference list

The references are an integral part of the manuscript and the most important thing is that the reference list must match the articles cited in the manuscript precisely and that all the necessary details of the references in the list must be complete and correct. Again please refer back to the Author Guidelines for referencing style and protocols.

The references that you do cite must be relevant and up to date. The latter does not mean that old references, in terms of dates, where absolutely necessary and relevant - cannot be cited. This would be particularly relevant in a systematic review of the literature. However, if there is up-to-date material that you are not citing in relation to the background to the study in particular, it suggests that you have not researched your evidence in any depth, nor read it or are biasing your argument by ignoring it. This is not good practice when writing articles for publication and reviewers will pick it up, as they are normally expert or experienced in the field they review (see Chapter 12).

Sometimes reviewers will suggest references to be read and cited as a result of this omission and often, although you will not be aware of this in the reviewing process, these may be the reviewer's own articles from the same specialist field. Sometimes editors will suggest articles and these may be from the journal you have submitted your manuscript to, and which again reflects on your weak preparatory reading.

Usually it is wise, simply, to cite these but do ensure that you have read them, that they are relevant and that you are citing them appropriately. Gratuitous citation of any articles should be avoided. If you do not think they are relevant then in your reply to reviewers on re-submission of an article you should state this, but most importantly, you must state why they are not relevant to the article in your opinion. It is important to do this as again the reviewers and editors are very supportive and contribute to the improvement of your paper; not to respond in any way is not good practice.

Citing your own work in an article is neither good nor bad practice, but it is common practice. This known as self-citation. If you are reporting work from a field where you have been active for many years, then it is natural that your own previous publications will be relevant and should be cited. In fact, you are doing yourself a disservice not to do this as you are omitting your own contribution to the field and the opportunity to have your article cited, which may contribute to your own citation record. The databases such as Web of Science (http://wok.mimas.ac.uk/) and Scopus (http://www.scopus.com/home.url), where people study citation patterns can easily distinguish between self-citation and citation by others to your work.

Software is now available to help you store references and to insert them into reference lists in the style of the journal you are writing for. Publishers encourage the use of such software as it tends to minimise errors in matching citations in the manuscript to the reference list and, as the references can be obtained and downloaded into the software directly from the Internet and databases, then it also minimises errors related to the accuracy of the references.

Appendices

Appendices are a matter of choice in a manuscript. Provided they are not included in the total word count then they are useful for providing additional information. They are also a useful place to present lengthy questionnaires if these are the subject of your article, or examples of interview questions. However, be aware of copyright issues here – ensure that the questionnaire is not already subject to copyright and seek permission to reproduce if it is. If the questionnaire is not subject to copyright and you have developed it, the copyright may then belong to the publisher. Increasingly, journals are asking for any additional material to be made available on the journal website and linked to the electronic version of the article and this may obviate the need for appendices. Readers can access the additional supplementary material by accessing the article online instead.

Better writing

Some specific poor aspects of your writing that editors will check and which you can learn to avoid will be covered in Chapter 11. Here, I will look at some general points that will help you to write better manuscripts. Some of this is related to the advice on getting started in Chapter 2.

The 'four rules' described in that chapter, as well as helping you get words onto the computer screen, will help your writing to flow. Therefore, in addition to setting and adhering to targets it is good, often, to use the first words that come to you mind while writing a section of a manuscript; in other words, do not struggle to find a more complicated or 'clever sounding' word – the one you write will usually be the right one. If not you can address this when you revise your draft manuscript. I often say to people: do not struggle to remember the word 'automobile' if you have written 'car'.

Writing in plain English

Nevertheless, if you write in this way and edit later – which is the recommended pattern – then you will often include words and phrases that are inappropriate and these should be replaced. You must not worry about this initially as, with practice, you will become better at getting it right first time. Therefore, avoid jargon and clichés. Jargon is language that only a few people, those familiar with that area of knowledge or 'in the know', will understand.

Jargon is much beloved of identifiable groups such as the armed forces and health professionals. It serves its purpose within the group but outside it leads to exclusion and confusion. You must write for as wide an audience as possible and assume a minimal knowledge of what you are writing about in all readers. You will rarely be criticised for writing plainly, but you will be criticised for writing that is not plain.

We hope that we have done this throughout the book, as it is not always a conscious activity when actually writing. This is why it pays to have your article read by a colleague prior to submission to a journal (see Chapter 2). Moreover, even within an identifiable group such as nurses, who exist worldwide, jargon does not transfer well across cultural and language barriers; therefore, write for an international audience. This is a key message for anyone writing in an international journal.

For example, from a UK perspective, how often do we refer among ourselves to 'SHAs' and 'PCTs' without realising that Strategic Health Authorities (SHA) and Primary Care Trusts (PCT) do not exist outside the United Kingdom? Even the NHS (National Health Service) has little currency outside the United Kingdom. Therefore, avoid using jargon, and even if you must refer in full to, for example, a Primary Care Trust, explain what it is. Clichés have no place in academic writing; they are commonly used phrases that are readily adopted by a wide range of people and, really, they are simply 'fillers' in conversation and, in fact, mean little or nothing.

Good examples are the football (soccer) managers' use of phrases such as 'at the end of the day'; 'the bottom line' and even worse examples. However, we all use clichés in our conversation; how often have you said that something has been 'swept under the carpet'? Usually, clichés can be replaced by a single word, for example 'at the end of the day' can be replaced by 'ultimately'; and 'swept under the carpet' can be replaced by 'ignored'. In the same vein, colloquial (common or familiar) language should be avoided; for example, 'kids' for 'children' and 'folks' for 'family'.

Losing words

One adage of good writing is that 'If it is possible to cut a word out, always cut it out' (http://www.pickthebrain.com/blog/george-orwells-5-rules-for-effective-writing/; Accessed 23 April 2012). You should try to use as few words as possible but you should not try too hard while you are writing: writing as you think and adding the additional word that helps you get to the next point can be a valuable way to write and to get words on the screen. However, you must revise your drafts, and one of the most valuable things you can do – and for someone else who asks you to revise their drafts – is to eliminate unnecessary words. The editor will also do this and I refer you to Chapter 11 for some specific examples. Meantime, I provide you with two examples of word reduction exercises in Boxes 5.13 and 5.14.

Box 5.13a Losing words exercise: concise writing: how to do it (long version)

It is becoming increasingly evident that clear, concise and parsimonious writing is an essential style to develop if you want to convey your ideas to other people using as few words as possible. In order to develop such a style it is necessary to follow a number of important steps. In order to become a concise writer you need, firstly, to write frequently and with regularity; secondly, it is essential to read your work closely and meticulously in order to eliminate unnecessary, extraneous and superfluous words; thirdly, it is essential to have another person read over your work carefully and meticulously in order to give you advice on where your style could be more concise and to correct any other aspects of your writing such as the structure of your sentences; your use of grammar, the extent to which your spelling is correct, the accuracy of information contained in what you have written and anything else that can improve the quality of what you have written (166 words).

The kind of things that you can eliminate by way of unnecessary and empty phrases include the use of '*in order*' as '*in order to do something*'; eliminating '*in order*' does not change the sense of the sentence and is more direct. Another common expression is 'a number of' which can easily be replaced by '*several*', '*some*' or '*a few*'. Using 'in which' is often replaceable by 'where' as in 'the hospital in which they worked' – use 'where'; sometimes, 'in which' can be eliminated as in 'the ways in which the nurses worked' – omit 'in which' and you have lost nothing.

If you read your work from this perspective you will quickly become adept at editing it and notice many things about your style of writing that can be altered; this is not the place to provide an exhaustive list but in a short time you will develop your own list of phrases to be eliminated or shortened.

Box 5.13b Losing words exercise: concise writing: how to do it (short version)

It is evident that clear and concise writing is essential if you want to convey your ideas using few words. To develop such a style you need to follow some important steps. To become a concise writer you need, first, to write frequently; second, you need to read your work meticulously to eliminate unnecessary words; third, it is essential to have another person read your work carefully to give you advice on your style and to correct other aspects such as the structure of sentences, grammar, spelling, the accuracy of information and anything else that can improve the quality of your writing. (102; 38% reduction)

A well-designed questionnaire is an essential aspect of any survey to make the survey more successful. The design of the questionnaire is important because the better the design of the questionnaire the better understood the questions in the questionnaire will be; this will make the answers to the questions better than if the questions were poorly written and it will also increase the return rate of the questionnaire. Questionnaires need to be designed for postal surveys, telephone surveys, face-to-face interviews and the World Wide Web. Whatever the type of questionnaire some basic essential rules apply: the questions need to be clearly written in the language which the questionnaire is being prepared; each question need to ask about one thing only otherwise people answering the questionnaire will not know which part of the question to respond to and if they do respond then the researcher will not know how to interpret the responses of the person responding to the questionnaire. Clearly, the presentation of a questionnaire designed to be used in a telephone or a face-to-face interview need not be designed to the same extent as one that is going to be sent out to people by post or that they are going to respond to on the Internet. For any type of questionnaire the questions need to be simple but for a postal survey the overall design of the questionnaire needs to be taken into consideration. Various different aspects of a questionnaire for a postal survey need to be taken into consideration including how clear the instructions for completing the questionnaire are; it needs to be considered how readable the questionnaire is and this takes into consideration points including the size of the font, the type of the font and the contrast of the font against the paper. Internet surveys are now very commonly used to gather data in surveys and there are several different online software packages available for the design and administration of Internet surveys (328 words).

Generally speaking, editors are good writers; they may not be experts on English grammar, but they usually know what is correct, acceptable and what works well. Common errors by authors in this regard include lack of agreement between singular and plural, for example 'the nurse liked their work' – here it should be 'the nurses liked their work' or 'the nurse liked his/her work'. Other things that editors will look out for is the correct use of phrases like 'compared to' which is often used when the author means 'compared with'. If two things are being compared, for example one nursing intervention with another then one is being compared 'with' the other – and this is usually what authors mean. If, on the other hand, one thing is being likened to another, for example, a new

A well-designed questionnaire is essential to any successful survey. The
design is important because the better the design the better understood
the questionnaire will be; this will make the answers to the questions better and increase the return rate. Questionnaires need to be designed for
postal, telephone, face-to-face interviews and the Internet. Whatever
the type of questionnaire some basic rules apply: the questions need
to be clearly written; each question need to ask one thing otherwise
respondents will not know which part of the question to respond to;
if they do respond then the researcher will not know how to interpret
the responses. The presentation of a questionnaire designed for telephone or a face-to-face interview need not be designed to the same
extent as one for a postal or Internet survey. For all questionnaires,
the questions need to be simple; for postal surveys, the overall design
needs to be considered. Various aspects of a postal survey questionnaire
need to be considered: including how clear the completion instructions
are; how readable the questionnaire is including font size and the contrast of the font against the paper. Internet surveys are now commonly
used to gather data, and several online software packages are available for the design and administration of Internet surveys (210 words;
37% reduction).

hospital was so luxurious that it was like a hotel then it would be compared
'to' a hotel and not with one.

It must be noted here that Editors do take account of those authors where
English is not their first language but it is advisable if this is you, then please
seek the guidance of someone who can help with translation and accuracy
of language or consider using translation services which some journals now
offer to help authors convey their research and innovation in a manner which
enhances the sharing of international scholarship.

Split infinitives and other things

There are some conventions that are based on the individual preference of
the editor and also some that are more or less acceptable, depending on which
side of the Atlantic you are writing for. Split infinitives – 'to otherwise think'
as opposed to 'to think otherwise' – the former has the split infinitive, is an
issue that has divided writers and editors for many years, with no resolution.
They are definitely more common and acceptable in the United States than
the United Kingdom, although some UK editors tolerate them. There are times
when it makes little difference; for example *'The objective of the exercise was*

to critically appraise the literature.' and *'The objective of the exercise was to appraise the literature critically.'*

This is not an issue that you should be overly concerned with when actually writing your article; however, understanding the issue may help to explain to you why changes have sometimes been made to your writing or if an editor asks for this issue to be addressed in your revised manuscript. Other preferences that also differ across the Atlantic are the use of the 'Oxford comma' in lists; in the United Kingdom it is conventional to separate lists of items with a comma, except the last item; for example *'the questionnaire included items on gender, age and occupation'* which, in the USA would read *'the questionnaire included items on gender, age, and occupation'*. Again, not something to be too concerned about in your writing pre-submission and any discrepancies from preferred style will be fixed at the production stage.

Submitting your manuscript

Once you have completed your manuscript you are ready to submit it and this is invariably done via the Internet. While the online submission systems such as Scholar One (http://scholarone.com/), the system used by Elsevier, for example see *International Journal of Nursing Studies* (http://ees.elsevier.com/ijns/) and the one used by Springer, for example, see *Quality of Life Research* (http://www.editorialmanager.com/qure/) are quite easy to use, they all have different features and it takes time to ensure that you have completed each step. Therefore, leave plenty of time to submit a manuscript, do not leave this until the end of the working day. If unsure about electronic submission then it is advisable to contact the editorial office or some journals even have tutorials online to show you how to access these and what to do when you get there. Some international and regional journals will still not have such systems in place and may still be requesting submitted articles via traditional means such as the postal service and sending in their article on a CD-ROM. Others may simply email their submission to the journal administrator. Whichever way you are required to do this ensure that you have kept an original copy and most importantly submitted the latest version of the article.

Conclusion

This chapter has covered the essential ingredients of a typical original article for an academic journal. The advice provided should apply to a wide range of journals and types of article. However, there is no substitute for reading the author guidelines for each journal you intend to submit to and also reading examples of the type of manuscript you intend to submit. It is hoped that by reading the three sections of this chapter that you now feel more confident both to write an article and to submit it for publication.

References

Darbyshire, P. (2004) 'Rage against the machine?': nurses' and midwives' experiences of using computerized patient information systems for clinical information. *Journal of Clinical Nursing*, 13, 17–25.

Long, T. & Fallon, D. (2007) Ethics approval, guarantees of quality and the meddlesome editor. *Journal of Clinical Nursing*, 16, 1398–1404. In *Journal of Clinical Nursing*, 17, 1534–1535.

Watson, R. (2006) Writing an abstract. *Nurse Author & Editor*, 16: 4. Available at: http://www.nurseauthoreditor.com/searchres.asp?cat=AUTHORS&page=4 [Accessed 23 April 2012] (Log in details required for direct access to this resource).

Watson, R. (2010) What's in a title? *Journal of Clinical Nursing*, 19, 2–3.

Chapter 6
Writing for Publication: The Book

Karen Holland

School of Nursing, Midwifery and Social Work, University of Salford, Salford, UK

Introduction

Writing a book is one of the most challenging writing for publication experiences. Although there are principles of writing that are similar to other forms of publication, writing a book has very different stages to it. In this chapter these will be explored through personal experiences and tips on good practice (and otherwise) in getting a book from first ideas to actual publication and sales of the book. It is worth noting that the majority of book authors do not earn much money from academic books, unless, for example, their book is adopted as a core text every year in curricula throughout the world.

Why write a book?

Most of us who write books, like myself and my co-editor, as well as some of our chapter authors, generally begin with an idea that a certain topic would be good for a book or, as in my first ever attempt (Holland and Hogg, 2001), the idea for the book came about as a result of the lack of key UK textbooks available for a module we were delivering in the area of trans-cultural nursing and cultural issues generally. This was a rapid learning experience, but it prepared me well for future attempts. Since that time other books have appeared on the UK market and we were invited to undertake a second edition of the book (Holland and Hogg, 2010), updated to accommodate changes in social policy and healthcare and cultural content, such as the issues around refugees and asylum seekers. This was very rewarding, as we knew the book still had a place in supporting students and colleagues in understanding and making a difference to the care of patients and their families, as well as colleagues from multi-cultural communities.

Writing for Publication in Nursing and Healthcare: Getting It Right, First Edition.
Edited by Karen Holland and Roger Watson.
© 2012 John Wiley & Sons, Ltd. Published 2012 by John Wiley & Sons, Ltd.

Therefore, for many of us, the ideas do start from a passion to make a difference, but also can be one where we wish to share our experiences and expertise with others to make a change in their professional careers; either undergraduate pre-registration students or for continuing professional development. This essentially was the rationale behind the development of this book, where both of us as editors of international peer-reviewed journal, who regularly engaged in writing for publication workshops, were now being asked for more than just helping someone get a paper published in a journal.

Getting started

There must first be an idea of the topic you are considering for a published book and what you might consider as research into what is currently around, for the audience you wish to write for, together with the messages/content you wish to convey. This is good practice if you are going to approach a publisher with the idea initially and then develop into a full book proposal (see Box 6.1 for example of book proposal requirements). If the publisher approaches you, having either been advised that you could write a book on a topic because of your expertise in a particular field, for example, then it is a different proposition and the discussion that ensues from that kind of initial approach will be different. Publishers also offer opportunities for academic staff in particular to talk to them at their workplace about ideas they may have and this offers another opportunity to explore ideas about potential books. You then have to choose between publishers.

Regardless of how you start, it is essential that once you have an idea, you talk it through either with a colleague, who may also be an excellent co-author, or an editor and do a background check of what is already available for your intended readership. In my experience it is important, though not an exact science, to consider the future possibilities for books, especially given the time frame involved between getting the idea, writing a proposal, persuading a publisher that the book is needed and would be a 'best-seller' and actual publication. For example, writing a book about social policy for nurses based on current issues without considering what the potential impact that these could have by the time the book is published and not including any chapters considering this would be an example of not thinking ahead. Of course, we are talking about academic/practice-focused books here and not ideas for writing a best-seller like J.K. Rowling and her Harry Potter books.

The ideas for a book, therefore, come from your own experience and interests, teaching and research activities, clinical practice developments and specific clinical skills, new areas such as service user engagement in nursing and a myriad of other issues that you encounter in your working day. For the purpose of this chapter I shall consider that you have an idea for a book and examine the steps involved in the process of getting that idea into a potential published book, while noting in different sections exceptions in relation to the other scenarios mentioned of how you got started on the challenging but rewarding journey.

Contacting a publisher

As this is a book being published by Wiley-Blackwell, I shall use their excellent Author Services as a point of reference for each stage of the publication process. Access to this can be found at: *http://authorservices.wiley.com/bk_authors.asp* and also their excellent comprehensive guide to preparing new book proposals: *http://authorservices.wiley.com/guidelines.asp*.

If you have an idea for a book it is prudent to begin by contacting the Commissioning Editor, who is responsible for commissioning books for publication. Their details can normally be accessed from similar sites to the aforementioned on different publishers' websites. The Commissioning Editor is also the person who will visit university departments to talk to staff about potential ideas for books. Communicate with them initially about your ideas, which is what we did for this book, and at same time agree to send a draft plan of what your ideas are.

Preparation is essential and will contribute to the discussion you have with the publishers and also demonstrate that you have thought clearly about the book proposed. The more homework you have done about their requirements, as in Box 6.1, the better it will be in trying to convince a publisher that the proposal is valid and will attract readers.

Activity 1

Consider from your own reading and book preference, what attracted you in the first place to wanting to read the book. Was it a necessity for a course you were undertaking or was it simply one that you had heard about, maybe read an abstract about it or obtained an inspection copy of it, which led to you purchasing it for yourself?

For most of us, buying academic textbooks usually means we are undertaking a course of study where the subject content of the book or books is relevant to the module outcomes. Alternatively, you could be a module leader who has to consider books for the module reading list and are faced with many different authored books on the subject, but in fact the content is the same or packaged differently.

Placing yourself in the situation of the possible reader of your book ideas can often help clarify your thinking about the focus and content of the book you wish to write. It can also be that you can see ahead a little – considering the kind of book that will be required for the future. Not an easy task but one that some authors do manage to envisage. The purpose of writing the book is therefore a key to developing your proposal, as is the audience for whom it is intended.

Writing a book proposal

When your ideas are more advanced and you have considered the rationale and development of the book, you can now submit a book proposal (see Box 6.1 for an example of the basics that most publishers require in an actual book proposal). Many publishers will have pro formas that you can download and complete online.

> **Box 6.1** Basic guideline for book proposal (Wiley-Blackwell 2011. http://authorservices.wiley.com/bk_authors.asp [accessed 12 October 2011])
>
> (1) *Overview*: A summary (200-300 words) of the book's aims and scope.
> (2) *Contents*: A contents list with a short paragraph describing each chapter.
> (3) *Readership*: A realistic assessment of the intended readership. Please try and be specific and stress the major markets. Consider the following:
>   (a) What level is it pitched (aimed) at?
>   (b) If applicable, for which course(s) will it be used? Will it be required for supplementary reading?
>   (c) Is its appeal international or confined to a particular geographical market?
> (4) *Competing titles*: A description of the book in relation to competing titles. This should include the following:
>   (a) The author, title, publisher, publication date, price and number of pages of the main competing titles
>   (b) Any unique features that will distinguish your book from the competition
> (5) *Other relevant information*:
>   (a) Your timetable: what stage are you at now? And when do you hope to complete the manuscript?
>   (b) How long is the final manuscript likely to be? That is, the number of words.
>   (c) How many line diagrams and photographs will there be?
>   (d) Will there be any unusual text features, such as colour or fold-outs?
> (6) *About the author(s)/editor(s)*: Please provide some brief information about yourself and co-authors, where appropriate, including any details of previous publications.

> ### Activity 2
>
> The best way of finding out if there is a need for a book in your area of interest as well as enabling you to consider the possibilities of writing one, is to use the template provided and test it out for yourself. Discuss with a colleague and determine whether you would, on the basis of what we will discuss next in relation to time and so on, wish to contact a publisher with your ideas.

Writing on your own: key issues to consider

It will be apparent to you from using the library or buying books that authorship varies from single authored books to those that have multiple editors and authors. Whatever the reason for writing a book, writing on your own can be a daunting but not insurmountable task. We all have our own way of doing things and sometimes we may wish to write a book that is not influenced by others' way of thinking, due possibly to the specific topic of the book itself or simply because that is the way you prefer to work. If you do decide to write on you own the same principles apply with regard to how you manage the whole of the task and it is a good idea to use the same principles of 'project management', such as a schedule of work, potential risks to completion and regular reports to the publisher.

Working on your own, however, does not mean that you do not discuss it with someone. As with any writing (Chapter 5) it is good practice to have your work peer reviewed, and there are some publishers who actively manage this through their own reviewer panel, some of whom may have been involved in review of the original proposal. From personal experience I have found this to be very helpful, particularly if your book is aimed at the student reader and there is an opportunity for student feedback on the book chapter content. Writing on your own could also involve writing a chapter in a book, often at the invitation of the editor who believes that your expertise in a subject would make a valued contribution to the book as a whole.

Writing with others: key issues to consider

Writing with others could mean either a joint editor role (as in this book) or writing a book chapter with a colleague (as evident in this book). Unlike writing a book on your own, you now have to consider how to work with others and it is essential from the beginning that everyone understands their role in writing their contribution to the overall book.

If you adopt an editor's role, you have the responsibility to the publishers to manage the book development and writing from chapter authors and deliver a complete manuscript on time. You may also have agreed to write a chapter or two in the book itself and managing your writing time and editor role can become a challenge. As with any writing, however, good planning and regular planned writing time is essential (Chapter 5). You will have signed a contract with the publishers if they choose to go ahead with the proposal you submitted. It is important to alert the publishers if you believe that you will need more time to submit the manuscript and some re-negotiation may be required as to the final deadline.

The process of writing a book: key issues to consider

Once you have had your proposal accepted then reality arrives in several forms, the main one being time to complete it. From a publisher's perspective, they have deadlines to meet once a book is commissioned. It is important that books are going to be published in time for new groups of students, especially when there has been a major change in curriculum needs, such as the Nursing and Midwifery Council (NMC) review of pre-registration nursing education that has led to all programmes throughout the United Kingdom from 2013 being at graduate degree at exit. Books, however, are not like an article, which can be written, revised and accepted for publication and published in the same year. To help those of you who may be considering writing a book, here are some tips, which we hope will help you with writing and managing the process.

Tips for successful management of writing a book

(1) If writing for student nurses, midwives or other healthcare professions, write for them and not yourself. This may seem a very odd statement but from experience and from discussing with other book authors and publishers, a book can be either an information giving one or a more interactive one in terms of the potential reader. For example if you were to write a book aimed at helping students learn to undertake leadership and management skills and practice, then a book just outlining theories of the subject, followed by information on different kinds of situations they might meet and possibly offering choices of what they might do would no doubt be helpful to them in terms of evidence base for their practice in leadership and management of patient care.

Imagine, however, that along with this approach that you also included student-focused scenarios from real life stories or reflections from other students or newly qualified nurses. How do you think a student in the third year of their programme undertaking the module on leadership and management in preparation for qualifying as a nurse might respond to the book?

Linking the theory and evidence base with the reality of practice situations not only helps the student understand the value in knowing why something is done but also enables them to problem solve in similar situations, which they might encounter for themselves.

(2) If writing for qualified nurses, the content might be similar but now the readership is practice based and already in a position of leadership and management. Therefore, they would need a book of a different kind, which focused not only on the rationales for undertaking certain management decisions but also an additional inclusion of topics on accountability as a qualified nurse.

(3) Planning of each step of the process in terms of time to write, holidays, work pressures and family needs must be built in, together with an element of risk management. Although this latter issue is unpredictable in terms of personal circumstances, which have to be managed at the time, other aspects mentioned can be factored in to the planning of the book. Often this has had to be agreed with the publisher, with some requiring regular drafts to be submitted and then being sent out to review on an continual basis, while others just need to be kept informed at set periods of the progress of the writing and ask to be alerted if possible changes have to be made to the time schedule of the completed manuscript.

Activity 3

If you have already written a book then it would be helpful to share your experiences with colleagues considering doing this. Decide what were the major challenges of your book writing experience and reflect on how you managed to overcome or manage these.

If you are about to embark on writing a book think about possible outcomes before you submit your proposal to the publisher, so that they can see that you have been realistic in your expectations as well as being good at planning for various options. Discuss with them at the pre-planning stage what you have to consider, especially if they wish to commission the book proposal for publication.

Remember we all started out writing books from a novice position and that despite experience in writing books in either an editor, co-author or single author role, none of us can plan for everything.

(4) It is important as you are writing the book or contributing a chapter to keep copies of your work to ensure that it is not lost. This does not mean that you have to print everything each time you make changes, but from experience it is worth saving work to different types of files, electronic being the main format. As soon as you have a completed a chapter (if an author in an edited book) or you are sent a completed chapter by an author (if editor of the book), it is in my experience a good idea to have at least one hard copy for filing. This is, however, often a personal preference rather than the rule.

(5) When writing a book it is essential that the readership is considered, especially if it is anticipated that the book could be read and used in different countries (see Box 6.1 – Wiley-Blackwell guide for authors). If the book is to be written for the international market then it has to written in a specific and general way rather than adopt a more ethnocentric view of the world. The evidence base, as well as possible exemplars from practice, has to be such that a reader in Australia or Japan will be able to understand the meaning and the context. This is probably the hardest aspect of writing a book, and some topics are more suited for an international audience than others.

Activity 4

Consider from your experience which book or books are more applicable to this universal language and content? Imagine you are accessing a well-known online shopping site and are searching for a book on a certain topic. You are faced with ten books on the subject from different countries. Which one do you choose?

If your book is on nursing practice, especially for undergraduate students, the majority of key texts are aimed at specific healthcare contexts and language fits in to this – an example being writing a book for the UK student and the NMC Standards and competencies and expecting it to be relevant to the student in the United States. There may be similarities in the actual art/science of nursing itself, but the actual clinical and educational context is nothing like this. The adoption of books transferred or translated into a different national context can actually work if translated correctly for content, but at the same time there may be situations where UK students are not allowed to undertake certain clinical skills pre-qualifying but those in the United States might. Caution is required if translating one book to another context. One field where writing across countries is less problematic is a research textbook, where the language of the content can be understood because the focus of the book can be considered universal.

Tips for being a book editor and author

Although the focus of this chapter is about considering good practice and principles of writing a book, for some of you this also may include undertaking the editor role, that is the person who will take responsibility for ensuring all the chapters have been written to a high standard and within an agreed time frame. A brief insight into this dual role may help those of you who have chosen to do this. Some key issues to consider are:

(1) What happens if an author of a chapter in a book you are editing is no longer able to write the chapter?

(2) What happens if your personal circumstances change suddenly?

(3) What happens if you are the editor of a book and the chapter authors you have asked to write a chapter and agreed have not adequately written to the standard you expected?

These are some of the outcomes that we have come across in our book publishing careers. If we consider them as unexpected risks then we can consider how we might manage them. The first one is not uncommon but obviously if you are the editor of a book and depending on when the commissioned author informs you, you will either have to find another author who can meet the deadlines set or have to write the chapter yourself for the same reason.

If the second option and your personal circumstances change, then if you are a co-editor with others then this is less problematic as someone can be asked to help out and take on a 'leadership' role temporarily or permanently. The third one is probably the most difficult to manage, especially if the authors are work colleagues. However, if the process of writing chapters and continual communication has taken place between everyone then this situation may have already been highlighted and help given to the author with writing the chapter to meet the expectations of the publisher and the editor or co-author. It is important that whatever role you have in writing a book for publication there is effective communication at the outset and also during the project itself.

What comes next?

The book is now written and sent to the publishers (in whatever format the publisher deems necessary such as electronic submission, CD-ROM and accompanied by a hard copy of the chapters as well) for copy editing (checking grammar, structure, references and a range of other text issues). Following the query stage and any corrections, the book is then returned to you at the proof stage to check everything is correct, that tables labelled correctly, names are correct, work is acknowledged and all permissions for use of material where appropriate has not only been sought but also noted in the book chapters. This latter issue is very important, as in article publication. The Wiley-Blackwell guidance has an excellent section on this issue of permissions.

Proofs are corrected (easier to check if more than one of you to ensure nothing major is missed) and returned to the publisher and production team. The covers of the book will have been chosen during this time as well, the editors having an input into this decision-making as we have in this book. Then the big day arrives and a copy of your book arrives at your office or home. The response to this will vary from author to author but from a personal viewpoint this has always brought a sense of achievement, and of course seeing and reading a copy belies none of the effort that has gone into both the writing and the editing of it.

Summary

Writing a book is a challenge, but for those of you who choose to do this, it can be a very rewarding one especially when you see colleagues and students reading and using it as a source of evidence and guidance for their own challenging journey of learning. If you are considering writing a book we hope that the information offered in this chapter and others in the book, which compliment this one, will enable you to consider various opportunities and options available to you. We wish you success with your endeavours.

References

Holland, K. & Hogg, C. (2001) *Cultural Awareness in Nursing and Health Care*, 1st edition. London: Arnold Publishers.

Holland, K. & Hogg, C. (2010) *Cultural Awareness in Nursing and Health Care*, 2nd edition. London: Arnold Publishers.

Websites

Wiley-Blackwell website for all information for authors or potential authors. Available at: http://authorservices.wiley.com/bk_authors.asp [Accessed 12 April 2012]. A specific one for preparing new book proposals. Available at: http://authorservices.wiley.com/guidelines.asp [Accessed 12 April 2012].

Sigma-Theta Tau: Book proposal instructions. Available at: http://www.nursingsociety.org/Publications/Books/Pages/BookProposal.aspx [Accessed 12 April 2012].

Chapter 7

Writing for Publication: The Essential Literature Review

Zena Moore

Faculty of Nursing and Midwifery, Royal College of Surgeons in Ireland, Dublin, Ireland

Introduction

Changes in the traditional, autocratic role of the doctor, combined with a better informed consumer have led to a more questioning approach to care delivery (Muir Gray, 2000). These changes demand of the health service increasing accountability, efficiency and effectiveness within available resources (Muir Gray, 2000). Therefore, those wishing to justify continued investment in current practice, or conversely, development of new innovative methods of care delivery, are expected to be explicit in their requests (Muir Gray, 2000). This explicitness has to include evidence-based material to support arguments appropriately (Muir Gray, 2000). Fundamentally, the emphasis on evidence-based practice (EBP) today has emerged due to changes in health service delivery, including greater emphasis on value for money, risk management, patient empowerment and the ever expanding role of information technology (Trinder, 2000).

The cornerstone of EBP is the integration of high-quality research evidence into clinical decision-making. This evidence is used in combination with clinical judgement and experience to plan the most appropriate patient treatment (Sackett et al., 1996). The applicability of research for clinical practice will depend on its quality (Sackett et al., 1996). Poorly conducted research will only yield poor results, which have no place in the clinical arena (Higgins and Altman, 2008b). It is argued that EBP comprises five main components: (1) identifying a clinical problem; (2) finding the evidence to answer the problem; (3) critically appraising the; evidence, (4) applying the evidence to the clinical situation; and, finally, (5) evaluating the results of the intervention (Reynolds, 2000). Central to this process is the identification of research that is of sound methodological quality, and critically appraising its merits or limitations (Sackett et al., 1996).

The purpose of conducting a literature review is to identify what is known and not known about a particular subject. In doing so, the authors attempt to summarise a body of literature, however, may not summarise the entire literature pertaining to the subject (Moore and Cowman, 2008a). A systematic review aims to summarise all the evidence available, published and unpublished, pertaining to a specific healthcare issue (Moore and Cowman, 2008a). For both the literature review and the systematic review, the information gained may be used in several ways, for example to support the current methods of care delivery, to act as the basis for changes in care delivery, to justify the need for investment in clinical practice or as a background providing the rationale for a particular research direction (McCarthy and O'Sullivan, 2008).

This chapter will focus on how to write a literature review or systematic literature review for publication in a journal. An introduction and recap on what is required for a review will initially be considered to establish clearly the difference between what constitutes a systematic review from one that is not as systematic, yet offers valued evidence in a specific field and is nonetheless rigorous in its critique of the evidence available. Both of these are important to specific fields but, as noted previously, the systematic review is one where all the literature on a topic has been evaluated, and the evidence provided can actually contribute to either a change in clinical practice as a result or a change in education or management practice. Learning how to write an effective systematic review is critical for those of you who may wish to publish aspects of a doctoral study, or have undertaken funded research projects where the recommendations for change need to demonstrate a systematic approach to evidence searching.

Where do we start? Initially we will consider the issues as if you had not undertaken a review as part of any study or project but simply wished to demonstrate your understanding of the evidence available on a topic prior to the possibility of undertaking either a funded research project or postgraduate study and wished to share this in a published piece of work. It is worth noting that for many who have undertaken such activity, finding a systematic review of the literature in your field of study is considered a veritable 'gold mine' or excellent resource, because someone has already carried out a rigorous evaluation and critique of the evidence that underpins some of the project work that *you* are undertaking. In understanding the stages of undertaking an actual review itself, you will be better able to consider writing your critical analysis of the findings for publication in a journal.

Decide the question/aims/objectives

Formulating the exact question/problem that needs to be addressed in the literature review can be a challenge (Murphy and Cowman, 2008). However, to identify the appropriate literature that will form the basis of the review, it is important to be clear about the research problem (Murphy and Cowman, 2008). Without this clarity, relevant literature may be missed, resulting in a

Box 7.1 Example of a review aim 1 (Cameron et al., 2011)

The aim of the review was to identify student characteristics and strate-gies in research studies investigating retention (why students stay) as opposed to attrition (why students leave) in nursing and midwifery pre-registration programmes.

poorly conducted review from which little meaning can be taken. To avoid this, the exact question, aim and objectives of the review should be outlined (Moore and Cowman, 2008a). For example, the aim of a review by Cameron et al. (2011) is clearly outlined in Box 7.1. The authors, as you can see, sought to identify student characteristics and strategies in research studies investigating retention, as opposed to attrition, in nursing and midwifery pre-registration programmes.

Whereas, Palfreyman et al. (2010), as seen in Box 7.2, set out systematically to review the literature with the aim of examining the quality of life questionnaires used to measure the impact of venous ulceration and to evaluate their psychometric properties. What is clear from these two examples is that the scope of the reviews, including the type of literature sought, is explicit within the aims. Cameron et al. (2011) were interested in retention *not* attrition literature, and Palfreyman et al. (2010) were primarily interested in the psychometric properties of the quality of life questionnaires in venous ulceration. Being explicit, means that much unnecessary literature may be excluded. For example Palfreyman et al. (2010) were not interested in wounds of all aetiologies, rather their focal point was on studies related to venous ulceration. Thus, studies relating to pressure ulcers and diabetic foot ulceration were not of interest, meaning the review is very specific in its focus. But this has been made implicit at the outset. This is an example of good practice in conducting and then writing a literature review. Rees (2010, p. 151) identifies a useful formula developed by Sackett et al. (1996) for developing a research question, which focuses on an intervention, that is the PICO formula.

Box 7.2 Example of review aim 2 (Palfreyman et al., 2010)

The aim of this study was to critically examine questionnaires that have been used to assess the impact of venous ulceration on quality of life. In addition, it also sought to promote consideration of quality of life as an outcome to measure the impact of nursing care on patients.

This acronym PICO stands for:

P: *Population*; *those (patients/clients) who form the focus of the review.*
I: *Intervention*; *that is the treatment.*
C: *Comparison*; *with an alternative treatment or no treatment.*
O: *Outcome*; *the measurable way that success is measured.*

(Rees, 2010, p. 151)

This type of formula may not of course be relevant if you are undertaking a review for a research question that has no clear intervention.

Tip 1

When writing your completed review for publication it is important to make clear the strategy that you undertook for the literature (evidence) search.

Activity 1

Using the two examples, consider writing your own systematic review of the literature on a topic that you think requires a clearer evidence base than is currently published. Set out a clear and focused aim for your review. This can then be the basis of using this chapter to follow through the topic under investigation at every stage of the process.

Identify the search strategy

To ensure transparency in the outcomes of the review, the precise search strategy used to retrieve potential literature needs to be outlined (Murphy and Cowman, 2008). In essence, this means that the terms used, the databases employed, the limits applied and the outcomes of the search should be clearly identified (Murphy and Cowman, 2008). If this detail is visibly alluded to, it means that those reading the work may appreciate the strengths and limitations of the review, in terms of how and where the literature was identified. Furthermore, replicating the search strategy should mean that others may retrieve a similar body of literature (Murphy and Cowman, 2008).

It is important also, to make clear why certain literature was excluded; in doing this the risk of deliberate bias in literature selection may be avoided.

For example, Gilmartin (2011) in conducting a review of contemporary cosmetic surgery, outlined the search strategy as follows:

[T]he search terms were: 'cosmetic surgery', 'associated risks', 'regulation of cosmetic surgery', 'awful cosmetic operations' and 'medical tourism';
the search engines used were: Cumulative Index to Nursing and Allied Health Literature (CINAHL), Medical Literature Analysis and Retrieval System on-line (Medline) and British Nursing Index (BNI);
and the limits applied were: English language, from 1982 to 2009.

Clearly, reading this search strategy immediately tells the reader that the review is limited, in that potential papers in other languages are not included.

Activity 2

Using your own identified aim (from Activity 1), identify key words/search terms for undertaking the initial review and identify which databases you are going to use. Remember the points raised previously and that anyone reading this on publication will need to be assured that all possible evidence has been sought.

An example of a published systematic review related to writing for publication itself is: McGrail, M.R., Rickard, C.M. & Jones, R. (2006) Publish or perish: a systematic review of interventions to increase academic publication rates. *Higher Education Research & Development*, 25(1), 19-35. Check out their aims and databases used.

There are often practical and financial reasons why reviews are limited to one language (Murphy and Cowman, 2008). Despite these reasons, it is important that readers of the reviews note the search limitations, as this may have an impact on the robustness and, as such, the generalisability of the review findings. For example, Bardy et al. (2008), in their systematic review of honey uses and its potential value within oncology care, applied an exclusion criteria to papers not published in English. The challenge with this exclusion criterion is that it is reasonably possible that there are more relevant papers published in other languages. Conversely, Lo et al. (2008), in their systematic review of sliver-releasing dressings in the management of infected chronic wounds, included both English and non-English papers, yielding a more robust review.

The systematic reviews published in the Cochrane library, offer insight into how search strategies are put together, they also offer a clear audit trail on how articles were included and excluded (Moore and Cowman, 2008a). It is of value to become familiar with some of the published Cochrane reviews, in order to become more aware of the process of developing a search strategy, see for example, Moore and Cowman (2005) and Moore and Cowman (2008b).

> **Activity 3**
>
> Access the Cochrane Collaboration website: http://www.cochrane.org/ and consider its publishing policy on systematic reviews: http://www .cochrane.org/policy-manual/225-publication-versions-cochrane-revie ws-print-journals. If you have access to Athens databases you can also access full texts of published reviews: http://www.thecochranelibrary .com/view/0/index.html.
>
> Consider the essential issues that you would have to consider to pub- lish a Cochrane type systematic review, including if any bias identified.

Identifying bias in the literature

The appraisal of evidence is the key to determining its relevance for clinical practice. The purpose of which is to identify the strengths and limitations of the included pieces of work. The critique forms the underlying thread run- ning through the review, as the review will summarise the evidence letting the reader know where the body of evidence lies (Moore and Cowman, 2009). However, in attempting to appraise and summarise the evidence, it is impor- tant to be aware of the variety of ways in which bias manifests itself in the literature. The Cochrane Collaboration defines bias as:

> *Something that will cause a consistent deviation from the truth.*
>
> *(Deeks et al., 2002, p. 2)*

This definition clearly identifies the challenges readers may have in inter- preting the clinical significance of research studies. Ultimately, the goal is to determine whether or not the methods employed in the study are reliable, valid or rigorous and, furthermore, are applicable to the specific clinical situation (Egger et al., 2001b).

A study is said to be valid when the researcher is using the right people for the study and measuring outcomes with the right instruments, that is mea- suring what is supposed to be measured (Anthony, 1999). *Reliability* is said to exist when the results achieved are consistent, that is if the researcher took the measurement more than once, the results would be the same (Anthony, 1999). Reliabilty does not imply validity; a clock may give the time consistently, but the time may be incorrect, that is it may be always 15 minutes fast (An- thony, 1999). Qualitative researchers do not tend to use the words reliability and validity; rather favour the use of the *concept of rigour* (Tobin and Begley, 2004). *Rigour* is the means by which the integrity of the research process in qualitative research is demonstrated and involves providing sufficient infor- mation to the reader such that the research may be replicated and similar findings achieved (Tobin and Begley, 2004).

There are multiple ways bias may manifest itself in the literature (Egger et al., 2001a). Publication bias is considered a problem when the authors of a study decide to publish or not publish research findings depending on whether the results are favourable or not (Egger et al., 2001a). Indeed, a systematic review by Hopewell et al. (2009) identified that trials with positive findings were more likely to be published than trials with negative or null findings. The authors would expect 41% of negative trials to be published. Conversely, 73% of positive trials would be expected to be published (Hopewell et al., 2009). It is important to be aware of non-significant findings, as having only some of the information will result in bias in interpreting the strength, or direction, of the evidence base, possibly leading to inappropriate conclusions to the review (Moore and Cowman, 2008a).

Time-lag bias can cause issues in determining the strength of evidence for or against a particular intervention (Egger et al., 2001a), as it is known that non-significant research findings take longer to appear in the literature (Misakian and Bero, 1998). A systematic review by Hopewell et al. (2007) found that trials with statistically significantly positive results in favour of the treatment under investigation were published in approximately 4–5 years. Conversely trials that were not statistically significant or were statistically significantly in favour of the control arm were published after 6–8 years (Hopewell et al., 2007). The implications of this for those undertaking literature reviews, is that they may unwittingly summarise the evidence in favour of the treatment under review, because of a lack of knowledge regarding the full extent of the evidence.

Even when undertaking a literature review that does not demand the same expectations as a Cochrane systematic review, there is still a need to be systematic in approaching the evidence base. Many authors who submit articles of their literature reviews to a journal often do not demonstrate understanding and critique of the evidence base they require for assuring confidence in their findings. This may to some extent be related to the word limitations of the journal itself, but by stating it is a review there is an expectation that key literature will have been identified and reviewed.

Activity 4

Obtain a copy of the following article and use it to support your endeavour to write a review for publication in a journal. It offers a broad overview of the key elements of a review article necessary for publication in a journal.

Green, B.N., Johnson, C.D. & Adams, A. (2001) Writing narrative literature reviews for peer-reviewed journals: secrets of the trade. *Journal of Sports Chiropractic and Rehabilitation*, 15, 5–19 (http://www.ncbi.nlm.nih.gov/pmc/articles/PMC2647067/pdf/main.pdf; Accessed 2 December 2011.)

A further issue regarding bias is citation bias, where the authors include or exclude publications for citation, depending on the direction of the results (Egger et al., 2001a; Nieminen et al., 2006). In other words, when conducting a literature review, the authors cite studies based on their *p*-value rather than their actual methodological quality (Nieminen et al., 2007). Citation bias alters the apparent direction of the research evidence, misleading the reader to conclude that there is greater weight of evidence in favour of a treatment than there is (Nieminen et al., 2007).

For example Rossouw et al. (1990) noted, in their critique of a published review of cholesterol lowering after myocardial infarction, that inclusion bias led to a completely different meta-analysis than would have been achieved had other studies been included. Although one study that met the inclusion criteria was available, it was excluded from the original review; along with 11 other studies where the reviewers had no clear rationale for their exclusion. The initial review found in favour of hormone treatment, whereas, inclusion by Rossouw et al. (1990) of the omitted studies, demonstrated the opposite.

A further bias is outcome reporting bias (Egger et al., 2001a). This type of bias is said to occur when not all of the original recorded outcomes are published on the basis of the results of the trial, rather there is selection of a portion of the results. Smyth et al. (2011) investigated the frequency and reasons for outcome reporting bias in clinical trials. In almost all trials reviewed (15/16, 94%), this under-reporting resulted in bias. In nearly a quarter of trials (4/17, 24%), the 'direction' of the main findings influenced the investigators' decision not to analyse the remaining data collected (Smyth et al., 2011). The presence of outcome reporting bias is high and as such can affect the conclusions that may be drawn when reviewing the literature Smyth et al., 2011. Essentially, the problem lies in the fact that a different conclusion may be drawn if the whole body of knowledge was available (Moore and Cowman, 2008a).

It seems clear that the appraisal of scientific evidence is challenging, with many pitfalls apparent that may mask the true nature of the evidence. Fundamentally, there are two components to this problem; firstly, what is considered to be 'evidence' and secondly how should this 'evidence' be reported, in order that one may have confidence in what has been read.

Critically evaluating the literature

To provide a succinct summary of the chosen literature, each component of the published paper needs to be explored and critically appraised. McCarthy and O'Sullivan (2008) suggest that the use of generic criteria for evaluating the literature may be helpful. These criteria explore issues from the design, sample selection, data collection, data analysis and findings, among others. These criteria are usually available in templates and are useful to enable the reviewer summarise the key components and strengths and limitations of the studies in an easily accessible manner, avoiding the need to refer back to the original paper during the writing of the review. An example of such a template to evaluate qualitative and quantitative methodological studies can be seen in Holland and Rees (2010) accessible online at: http://www.oup.com/uk/orc/bin/9780199563104/01student/chapters/ch07/frameworks/ (Accessed 12 December 2011). Although these tools are aimed at mainly undergraduate students, they still remain a useful framework for criteria to be considered for a published review of the literature in either paradigm.

The Joanna Briggs Institute has a toolkit called RAPid: (see http://connect.jbiconnectplus.org/Appraise.aspx; Accessed 12 December 2011), which it states as:

> RAPid is designed to assist individual practitioners and undergraduate and postgraduate students to acquire the skills of posing relevant questions about the feasibility, appropriateness, meaningfulness or effectiveness of an intervention or professional activity, and to pursue this question through applying the following basic steps of the comprehensive systematic review process:
>
> Topic identification and rigorous question development
> Searching for the evidence
> Critically appraising the evidence
> Summarising the evidence
> Reporting the results of this process in an accessible format to maximise knowledge transfer to practice
>
> (The Joanna Briggs Institute)

Although use of generic templates for evaluating the literature are useful, there are some specific considerations in different research designs that warrant consideration and these will be discussed further. That is, in case this is what they want to write up – of course, it helps that they are also being told what to do first! Then they can have tips about what to include in their written-up review for different media – whether journal article or report, etc.

Assessing quality issues in randomised controlled clinical trials

The randomised controlled trial (RCT) is considered the gold standard for evaluating the effect of interventions used in clinical practice (Egger and Smith, 2001). RCTs are not the only form of evidence and the selection of the most appropriate methodology for a study will depend on the question being asked. The Cochrane Collaboration has several key issues that they consider important in the assessment of the quality and impact on the external validity of RCTs. These include randomisation, allocation concealment, baseline comparability, blinding and intention-to-treat (ITT) (Higgins and Altman, 2008b).

Randomisation

In an RCT the researcher is interested in determining the effect of a specific intervention on a group of participants; if one can determine with confidence, that any effects noted have occurred due to the intervention and not as a result of a specific characteristic of the participants in one of the study groups (Altman, 1991). The use of an experimental group and control group in the RCT determines the effects of intervention. However, depending on how groups are allocated to the specific arms of the study, bias can emerge.

Using random methods means that each and every participant has an equal chance of being allocated to either one or other of the study groups (Bland, 2000), thus preventing researcher bias when selecting participants or the group to which they are allocated (Altman, 1991). This is also important when one is wishing to infer back to the population from whom the sample was generated. Inferential statistical methods employed in a study are based on the premise that the sample has been selected using random methods (Altman, 1991). Without this criterion, the results are not applicable beyond the sample. Fundamentally, the importance of randomisation lies in its contribution to reducing bias, thereby enhancing the confidence that one may have in the results of a clinical trial (Schultz and Grimes, 2002).

Moher and colleagues (1998) explored the effect that the quality of reporting of clinical trials had on the effect 'estimates of intervention efficacy', reported in meta-analysis. They included 11 published meta-analyses that had been previously reported in either medical journals or the Cochrane Database of Systematic Reviews. Only 15% of the 127 studies included in the meta-analyses reported the methods used to generate the randomisation sequence. The average treatment effect was 52% for low-quality trials (OR 0.48 [0.43–54]). When adjusted for poor quality the treatment effects reduced to 35% (OR 0.65 [0.59–0.71]).

Allocation concealment

Allocation concealment is a randomisation method that prevents the researcher influencing which group, experimental or control, a participant is allocated to (Higgins and Altman, 2008b), rather ensuring that the participant is assigned to a specific study group by chance (Higgins and Altman, 2008b). Studies without adequate allocation concealment tend to report larger estimates of effect when compared to those who describe adequate allocation concealment (Schulz, 2000). Indeed, one study showed that in studies without adequate allocation concealment, there was a tendency to report an increased estimate of effect (37%; ROR = 0.63; 95% CI 0.45–0.88). This suggested that in the presence of lower quality trials, the treatment effect may be exaggerated, and this large margin of error needs to be considered in the interpretation of the outcomes of such studies. This has important implications for clinical practice where decisions regarding patient care may be made based on the results of these trials.

Baseline comparability

Baseline data refers to the data collected from each participant before beginning the trial (Friedman et al., 1996). This includes demographic information, medical condition and prognostic factors and where appropriate, socioeconomic information. This allows the researcher to determine if participants in both arms of the study are comparable at the outset of the study (Friedman et al., 1996) and allows those evaluating the study to determine if the characteristics of those participating in the study are similar to those normally encountered in the reader's clinical practice (Friedman et al., 1996). The external validity of the study is central in determining whether the findings are applicable in the clinical setting.

The randomisation process, if applied correctly, should ensure baseline comparability; that is, differences between the groups at baseline have occurred by chance (Pocock et al., 2002). However, there can be factors specific to certain patients that the researcher may be unaware of. Such factors may manifest themselves during the trial and sub-group analysis may clarify the statistical significance of such differences (Pocock et al., 2002). Interestingly, in a systematic review of pressure ulcer cleansing products (Moore and Cowman, 2005), two of the three trials included failed to provide adequate information pertaining to baseline comparability (Griffiths et al., 2001; Bellingeri et al., 2004) and one study did not provide any information pertaining to the baseline characteristic of the subjects (Burke et al., 1998). Similarly, in a review of therapeutic ultrasound for pressure ulcers (Baba-Akbari Sari et al., 2006), two of the studies reported baseline data (Nussbaum et al., 1994; ter Riet et al., 1995), whereas the third study did not report this information fully (McDiarmid et al., 1985). It appears, however, that those papers published more recently include more relevant information pertaining to baseline characteristics, suggesting that this component is now considered important in determining the quality of a clinical trial (Pocock et al., 2002).

Blinding

Blinding of the study is said to be complete if the investigators, the participants, the outcome assessor and the individual analysing the data have no idea which group the participant is allocated to (Higgins and Altman, 2008b). Human behaviour is influenced by prior knowledge, thus, without blinding, there is a risk that the size of the effect may be overestimated, resulting in a bias in favour of the treatment (Day and Altman, 2000). Therefore, blinding is considered important in the assessment of subjective outcomes, such as ease of use of a treatment, and in ensuring comparability of assessment and diagnostic interventions across all groups within a study (Higgins and Altman, 2008b). Fundamentally, the objective of blinding is to maximise the quality and believability of the data derived from a clinical trial (Bang et al., 2004). However, in a study by Fergusson and colleagues (2004), only 2% of 191 trials reported in the medical literature from 1998 to 2001 provided evidence of the success of blinding. Further, in another study, reports from un-blinded studies resulted in a 34% greater estimate of treatment effect (ROR = 0.66; 95% CI 0.52–0.83) (Moher et al., 1998).

Intention-to-treat

ITT analysis means that participants are analysed according to the group they were originally allocated to even if they do not adhere to the study protocol or complete the study. The rationale for using ITT analysis is two-fold; it maintains treatment groups that are similar (apart from random variation) and, therefore, validates the use of randomisation (Hollis and Campbell, 1999), and allows for handling of protocol deviations, further protecting the randomisation process (Hollis and Campbell, 1999). Essentially, omitting those who do not complete the study from the final analysis may bias the outcomes of the study, because those who do not complete may do so because of adverse effects of the intervention (Montori and Guyatt, 2001).

ITT analysis is considered one of the key quality indicators in any research study (Campbell et al., 2004). However, in three systematic reviews reported in the Cochrane library, it was not conducted or not reported in 2 of 3 studies (Moore and Cowman, 2005), 4 of 7 studies (Ubbink et al., 2008) and 17 of 19 studies (Jull et al., 2008). This suggests that this quality indicator has not yet been completely integrated into clinical research. The challenge with not including those who do not complete the study in the final analysis is that it suggests that those who adhere to the protocol tend to do better than those who do not comply (Montori and Guyatt, 2001). The risk is that the researcher will make a type 1 error, which is to reject the null hypothesis, when it is true (Lachin, 2000). Indeed, it is argued that the probability of committing a type 1 error increases by 0.50 in the absence of ITT (Lachin, 2000).

To place trial evidence on the correct rung of the hierarchy ladder, it needs to be appraised for the relative merits of results achieved. Fundamentally, individuals conducting critical appraisal are asking whether the study findings can be believed (Higgins and Altman, 2008a). To meet the challenge of reporting clinical trials in published literature, a group of experts developed the consolidated standards of reporting trials (CONSORT) statement, published in 1996 (Begg et al., 1996), which was later revised and published in 2001 (Moher et al., 2001). There are 22 items included in the CONSORT checklist, the purpose of which is to standardise the reporting of clinical trials and thus simplify the quality appraisal process (Moher et al., 2001). When appraising clinical trials it is a good idea to use the CONSORT statement to guide you in the areas you need to consider to determine the studies methodological rigor (see http://www.consort-statement.org/consort-statement/).

Assessing quality issues in qualitative studies

Assessment of quality issues in qualitative studies is not a straightforward process and many of the instruments used for clinical trials do not readily apply (Noyes et al., 2011). There are a wide variety of instruments available, all of which have been designed specifically for qualitative research. However, as such, there is variance among these instruments and a lack of consistency in approach may be a concern (Noyes et al., 2011). Despite these challenges, qualitative data have been analysed in a variety of different circumstances alone or alongside clinical trials, in a systematic manner, yielding valuable insights into individual's experiences (Noyes and Popay, 2007).

Horsburgh (2003) argues that the evaluation of qualitative research requires adoption of rigorous methods in order that the clinical implications of the findings may be determined. Furthermore, adoption of these rigorous methods is possible if, for example, the reviewer follows the guidance of Popay et al. (1998). These authors (Popay et al., 1998) suggest that there are three interrelated criteria that are the basis of good qualitative health research. These criteria are the following:

(1) Interpretation of subjective meaning, that is the participants' accounts is the basis upon which all the analysis and interpretation are clearly founded (Popay et al., 1998; Horsburgh, 2003).
(2) Description of social context, that is the study should provide clear background information about the environment in which the participants were situated (Popay et al., 1998; Horsburgh, 2003).
(3) Attention to lay knowledge, that is within a study the participants' own points of view and perspectives are given equal weighting to those of 'experts' in the field (Popay et al., 1998; Horsburgh, 2003).

What does this mean for someone wanting to write a review for publication? Consideration of these issues is important for you when reviewing qualitative literature, as they will help you determine the trustworthiness of the studies. This information is important to include in your review, so the reader may understand the strengths and limitations of the studies you have included.

Horsburgh (2003) adds some other criteria to consider, such as sampling. While acknowledging that sampling in qualitative research does not follow the same rigorous process as in qualitative research, nonetheless, the sampling should be adequate. In other words, does the sampling provide for the possibility of adequate exploration of the subject and the context in which the subject matter is located (Horsburgh, 2003)? A further criterion is flexibility, whereby there is variability rather than rigidity in the research approach. This is considered important to allow for the natural emergence of a change in direction based upon the continuous analysis of the data during the research process (Horsburgh, 2003).

Finally, Horsburgh (2003) argues that generalisability of findings is an important concern in qualitative research. However, it does not follow the probabilistic generalisability seen in quantitative research, rather it is a theoretical generalisability (Horsburgh, 2003). In other words, the research should explore the theoretical possibility that the theory developed in one study may be used to provide explanatory theory for the experiences of other individuals in similar circumstances (Horsburgh, 2003).

Write the review

Having critically appraised the literature, allowing the findings to emerge from what has been read, the next step is to write the review (McCarthy and O'Sullivan, 2008). It is important to have a good structure for how the review will flow, such that it follows a logical sequence of thought, which is easily understood by the reader (McCarthy and O'Sullivan, 2008). Presentation of a synthesis of the literature is the key to ensuring readability and clarity in presentation of the salient points (Aveyard, 2010).

Use of a mind map (Figure 7.1) to plan out the sections of the review is worthwhile, as this allows the writer logically plan out how the review will look (Heinrich, 2001). First, all the ideas that have arisen from what has been read should be written down; furthermore, these ideas should be linked to the congruent and divergent issues within the literature (Heinrich, 2001). These ideas are then linked to themes and emerging interconnecting themes are brought together (Heinrich, 2001). Following this, the rhetoric that supports the themes is added, including the arguments from the literature that support or refute the theme (Heinrich, 2001). Finally, the order that the themes should appear in the review is decided, ideally moving from the general to the specific (Heinrich, 2001).

Actually writing the review can be challenging, as the writer has to balance between the provision of sufficient information to enable understanding, with the exclusion of information considered unnecessary (Heinrich, 2001). The review should include a succinct overview of the methodological issues arising in the literature, such that the reader may appreciate the generalisability of the review findings (McCarthy and O'Sullivan, 2008). Furthermore, the recommendations made should be founded in the literature that has been read, with the gaps in current knowledge clearly identified (McCarthy and O'Sullivan, 2008). Fundamentally, the writer is attempting to provide a balanced,

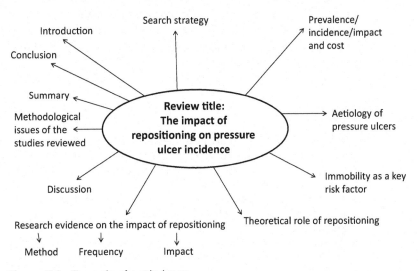

Figure 7.1 Example of a mind map.

unbiased review of what has been read in order to make recommendations for practice and future research.

> ### Activity 5
>
> If you have followed all the steps outlined in this chapter, as well as accessed the numerous resources and references highlighted throughout, it is pertinent now that you undertake to write either a literature review that is systematic in its approach to finding evidence on a topic, or a full systematic review as per Cochrane guidance.

You may have undertaken either one as a part of postgraduate studies or as a part of research project report for a funding body. Publishing a review of any kind is rewarding as well as being practical, as it gathers evidence together on a specific subject to enable you to make valid and reliable recommendations to those reading it.

Conclusion

The purpose of writing a literature review, whether it is called a systematic review or not, is to provide a summary of what is known and not known about a particular body of literature. In doing so the writer needs to be explicit about the review question, how the literature was searched and retrieved, including the rationale for non-inclusion of particular papers. In addition, the methods for critical appraisal of the literature should be clearly outlined, which should, ideally, follow a systematic, logical format. Writing the review can be challenging, but use of a mind map may be of assistance in lending clarity to the themes that should be included, in addition to the relevant supporting or refuting data emerging from what has been read. Finally, the recommendations made should be clearly linked to what has been read and presented, including the methodological challenges and limitations. The purpose of this is to guide practice and future research.

References

Altman, D. (1991) Clinical trials. In: Altman, D.G. (Ed.) *Practical Statistics for Medical Research*. Boca Raton, FL: Chapman & Hall/CRC, pp. 440-476.

Anthony, D. (1999) Validity and reliability. In: *Understanding Advanced Statistics*. London: Churchill Livingstone, pp. 29-44.

Aveyard, H. (2010) How do I synthesize my findings? In: Aveyard, H. (Ed.) *Doing a Literature Review in Health and Social Care*, 2nd edition. New York: McGraw Hill, pp. 123-140.

Baba-Akbari Sari, A., Flemming, K., Cullum, N.A. & Wollina, U. (2006) Therapeutic ultrasound for pressure ulcers. *Cochrane Database of Systematic Reviews*, CD001275.

Bang, H., Ni, L. & Davis, C.E. (2004) Assessment of blinding in clinical trials. *Controlled Clinical Trials*, 25, 143-156.

Bardy, J., Slevin, N., Mais, K. & Molassiotis, A. (2008) A systematic review of honey uses and its potential value within oncology care. *Journal of Clinical Nursing*, 17, 2604-2623.

Begg, C., Cho, M., Eastwood, S., Horton, R., Moher, D., Olkin, I., Pitkin, R., Rennie, D., Schulz, K.F., Simel, D. & Stroup, D. (1996) Improving the quality of reporting of randomized controlled trials. The CONSORT statement. *Journal of the American Medical Association*, 276, 637-639.

Bellingeri, R., Attolini, C., Fioretti, O., Forma, P., Traspedini, M. & Costa, M. (2004) Evaluation of the efficacy of a preparation for the cleansing of cutaneous injuries [Valutazione dell effcacia di un presido per la detersione delle lesioni cutanee - Studio multicentrico in aperto controllato e randomizzato]. *Minerva Medica*, 95, 1-9.

Bland, M. (2000) The design of experiments. In: *An Introduction to Medical Statistics*, 3rd edition. Oxford: Oxford University Press, pp. 5-25.

Burke, D.T., Ho, C.H.K., Saucier, M. & Stewart, G. (1998) Effects of hydrotherapy on pressure ulcer healing. *American Journal of Physical Medicine and Rehabilitation*, 77, 394-398.

Cameron, J., Roxburgh, M., Taylor, J. & Lauder, W. (2011) An integrative literature review of student retention in programmes of nursing and midwifery education: why do students stay? *Journal of Clinical Nursing*, 20, 1372-1382.

Campbell, M.K., Elbourne, D.R., Altman, D.G. & CONSORT group (2004) CONSORT statement: extension to cluster randomised trials. *British Medical Journal*, 328, 702-708.

Day, S.J. & Altman, D.G. (2000) Statistics notes: blinding in clinical trials and other studies. *British Medical Journal*, 321, 504.

Deeks, J., Higgins, J., Riis, J. & Silagy, C. (2002) Cochrane Collaboration open learning material for reviewers. The Cochrane Collaboration, Oxford. Available at: http://publicat.bham.ac.uk/46925/ [Accessed 20 June 2004].

Egger, M., Dickersin, K. & Smith, G.D. (2001a) Problems and limitations in conducting systematic reviews. In: Egger, M., Smith, G.D. & Altman, D.G. (Ed.) *Systematic Reviews in Health Care Meta-Analysis in Context*, 2nd edition. London: British Medical Journal, pp. 43-68.

Egger, M. & Smith, G.D. (2001) Principles of and procedures for systematic reviews. In: Egger, M., Smith, G.D. & Altman, D.G. (Eds.) *Systematic Reviews in Health Care Meta-Analysis in Context*, 2nd edition. London: British Medical Journal, pp. 23-42.

Egger, M., Smith, G.D. & O Rourke, K. (2001b) Rationale, potentials and promise of systematic reviews. In: Egger, M., Smith, G.D. & Altman, D.G. (Eds.) *Systematic Reviews in Health Care Meta-Analysis in Context*, 2nd edition. London: British Medical Journal, pp. 3-22.

Fergusson, D., Cranley Glass, K., Waring, D. & Shapiro, S. (2004) Turning a blind eye: the success of blinding reported in a random sample of randomised, placebo controlled trials. *British Medical Journal*, 328, 432-437.

Friedman, L.M., DeMets, D.L. & Furberg, C.D. (1996) Baseline assessment. In: Friedman, L.M., DeMets, D.L. & Furberg, C.D. (Eds.) *Fundamentals of Clinical Trials*, 3rd edition. Basel, Switzerland: Birkhäuser, pp. 130-139.

Gilmartin, J. (2011) Contemporary cosmetic surgery: the potential risks and relevance for practice. *Journal of Clinical Nursing*, 20, 1801-1809.

Griffiths, R.D., Fernandez, R.S. & Ussia, C.A. (2001) Is tap water a safe alternative to normal saline for wound irrigation in the community setting? *Journal of Wound Care*, 10, 407-411.

Heinrich, K. (2001) Mind-mapping: a successful technique for organizing a literature review. *Nurse Author & Editor*, 11, 4, 7-8.

Higgins, J.P.T. & Altman, D. (2008a) Assessing risk of bias in included studies. In: Higgins, J., Green, S. & Cochrane Collaboration (Eds.) *Cochrane Handbook for Systematic Reviews of Interventions*. London: John Wiley & Sons, pp. 187-243.

Higgins, J.P.T. & Altman, D.G. (2008b) Assessing risk of bias in included studies. In: Higgins, J.P.T. & Green, S. (Eds.) *Cochrane Handbook for Systematic Reviews of Interventions*. Version 5.0.0 (updated February 2008), Oxford. The Cochrane Collaboration available at: www.cochrane-handbook.org [Accessed 12 April 2012].

Hollis, S. & Campbell, F. (1999) What is meant by intention to treat analysis? Survey of published randomised controlled trials. *British Medical Journal*, 319, 670-674.

Hopewell, S., Clarke, M., Stewart, L. & J.T. (2007) Time to publication for results of clinical trials. *Cochrane Database of Systematic Reviews*, MR000011.

Hopewell, S., Loudon, K., Clarke, M., Oxman, A. & Dickersin, K. (2009) Publication bias in clinical trials due to statistical significance or direction of trial results. *Cochrane Database of Systematic Reviews*, MR000006.

Horsburgh, D. (2003) Evaluation of qualitative research. *Journal of Clinical Nursing*, 12, 307-312.

Jull, A.B., Rodgers, A. & Walker, N. (2008) Honey as a topical treatment for wounds. *Cochrane Database of Systematic Reviews*, CD005083.

Lachin, J.M. (2000) Statistical considerations in the intent-to-treat principle. *Controlled Clinical Trials* 21, 167-189.

Lo, S., Hayter, M., CJ, C., WY, H. & Lee, L. (2008) A systematic review of silver-releasing dressings in the management of infected chronic wounds. *Journal of Clinical Nursing*, 17, 1973-1985.

McCarthy, G. & O'Sullivan, D. (2008) Evaluating the literature. In: Watson, R., Mc Kenna, H., Cowman, S. & Keady, J. (Eds.) *Nursing Research: Designs and Methods*. London: Churchill Livingstone, pp. 113-123.

McDiarmid, T., Burns, P.N., Lewith, G.T. & Machin, D. (1985) Ultrasound in the treatment of pressure sores. *Physiotherapy*, 71, 66-70.

Misakian, A.L. & Bero, L.A. (1998) Publication bias and research on passive smoking: comparison of published and unpublished studies. *Journal of the American Medical Association*, 280, 250-253.

Moher, D., Jones, A., Cook, D.J., Jadad, A.R., Moher, M., Tugwell, P. & Klasse, T.P. (1998) Does quality of reports of randomised trials affect estimates of intervention efficacy reported in meta-analyses? *The Lancet*, 352, 609-613.

Moher, D., Schulz, K.F. & Altman, D. (2001) The CONSORT statement: revised recommendations for improving the quality of reports of parallel-group randomized trials. CONSORT group. *Journal of the American Medical Association*, 285, 1987-1991.

Montori, V.M. & Guyatt, G.H. (2001) Intention-to-treat principle. *Canadian Medical Association Journal*, 165, 1339-1341.

Moore, Z. & Cowman, S. (2008a) The Cochrane Collaboration, systematic reviews and meta analysis. In: Watson, R., Mc Kenna, H., Cowman, S. & Keady, J. (Eds.) *Nursing Research: Designs and Methods*. London: Churchill Livingstone, pp. 101-111.

Moore, Z. & Cowman, S. (2009) Nurses need critical appraisal skills when reading research. *Nursing Times*, 105, 33.

Moore, Z.E.H. & Cowman, S. (2005) Wound cleansing for pressure ulcers. *Cochrane Database of Systematic Reviews*, CD004983.

Moore, Z.E.H. & Cowman, S. (2008b) Risk assessment tools for the prevention of pressure ulcers. *Cochrane Database of Systematic Reviews*, CD006471.

Muir Gray, J.A. (2000) Evidence-based public health. In: Trinder, L. & Reynolds, S. (Eds.) *Evidence-Based Practice a Critical Appraisal*. Oxford: Blackwell Publishing Ltd., pp. 89–110.

Murphy, P. & Cowman, S. (2008) Accessing the nursing research literature. In: Watson, R., Mc Kenna, H., Cowman, S. & Keady, J. (Eds.) *Nursing Research: Designs and Methods*. London: Churchill Livingstone, pp. 75–87.

Nieminen, P., Carpenter, J., Rucker, G. & Schumacher, M. (2006) The relationship between quality of research and citation frequency. *BMC Medical Research Methodology*, 6, 42–49.

Nieminen, P., Rucker, G., Miettunen, J., Carpenter, J. & Schumacher, M. (2007) Statistically significant papers in psychiatry were cited more often than others. *Journal of Clinical Epidemiology*, 60, 939–946.

Noyes, J. & Popay, J. (2007) Directly observed therapy and tuberculosis: how can a systematic review of qualitative research contribute to improving services? A qualitative meta-synthesis. *Journal of Advanced Nursing*, 57, 227–243.

Noyes, J., Popay, J., Pearson, A., Hannes, K. & Booth, A. (On behalf of the Cochrane Qualitative Research Methods Group) (2011) Qualitative research and Cochrane reviews. In: Higgins, J. & Green, S. (Eds.) *Cochrane Handbook for Systematic Reviews of Interventions*. Version 5.1.0 (updated March 2011). The Cochrane Collaboration.

Nussbaum, E.L., Biemann, I. & Mustard, B. (1994) Comparison of ultrasound/ultraviolet-C and laser for treatment of pressure ulcers in patients with spinal cord injury. *Physical Therapy*, 74, 812–825.

Palfreyman, S., Tod, A., Brazier, J. & Michaels, J. (2010) A systematic review of health-related quality of life instruments used for people with venous ulcers: an assessment of their suitability and psychometric properties. *Journal of Clinical Nursing*, 19, 2673–2703.

Pocock, S.J., Assmann, S.E., Enos, L.E. & Kasten, L.E. (2002) Subgroup analysis, covariate adjustment and baseline comparisons in clinical trial reporting: current practice and problems. *Statistics in Medicine*, 21, 2917–2930.

Popay, J., Rogers, A. & Williams, G. (1998) Rationale and standards for the systematic review of qualitative literature in health services research. *Qualitative Health Research*, 8, 341–351.

Rees, C. (2010) Searching and retrieving evidence to underpin nursing practice. In: Holland, K. & Rees, C. (Eds.) *Nursing: Evidence-Based Practice Skills*. Oxford: Oxford University Press, pp. 143–166.

Reynolds, S. (2000) The anatomy of evidence-based practice: principles and methods. In: Trinder, L. & Reynolds, S. (Eds.) *Evidence-Based Practice a Critical Approach*. Oxford: Blackwell Publishing Ltd., pp. 17–34.

Rossouw, J.E., Lewis, B. & Rifkind, B.M. (1990) The value of lowering cholesterol after myocardial infarction. *New England Journal of Medicine*, 323, 1112–1119.

Sackett, D.L., Rosenberg, W.M.C., Gray, J.A.M., Haynes, R.B. & Richardson, W.S. (1996) Evidence-based medicine: what it is and what it isn't. *British Medical Journal*, 312, 71–72.

Schultz, F.K. & Grimes, D.A. (2002) Generation of allocation sequences in randomised trials: chance, not choice. *The Lancet*, 359, 515–519.

Schulz, K.F. (2000) Assessing allocation concealment and blinding in randomised controlled trials: why bother? *Evidence Based Medicine*, 5, 36–38.

Smyth, R., Kirkham, J., Jacoby, A., Altman, D., Gamble, C. & Williamson, P.R. (2011) Frequency and reasons for outcome reporting bias in clinical trials: interviews with trialists. *British Medical Journal*, 342:c7153. doi: 10.1136/bmj.c7153.

ter Riet, G., Kessels, A.G.H. & Knipschild, P. (1995) A randomized clinical trial of ultrasound treatment for pressure ulcers. *British Medical Journal*, 310, 1040-1041.

Tobin, G. & Begley, C. (2004) Methodological rigour within a qualitative framework. *Journal of Advanced Nursing*, 48, 388-396.

Trinder, L. (2000) Introduction: the context of evidence-based practice. In: Trinder, L. & Reynolds, S. (Eds.) *Evidence-Based Practice a Critical Appraisal*. Oxford: Blackwell Publishing Ltd., pp. 1-16.

Ubbink, D.T., Westerbos, S.J., Evans, D., Land, L. & Vermeulen, H. (2008) A systematic review of topical negative pressure for treating chronic wounds. *Cochrane Database of Systematic Reviews*, 95(6), 685-692.

Further reading

Bettany-Saltikov, J. (2010) Learning how to undertake a systematic review: Part 1. *Nursing Standard*, 24(50), 47-55.

Hart, C. (2003) *Doing a Literature Review*, London: Sage Publications.

Henderson, L.K., Craig, J.C., Willis, N.S., Tovey, D. & Webster, A.C. (2010) How to write a Cochrane Systematic Review. *Nephrology*, 15, 617-624.

Holland, K. & Rees, C. (2010) *Nursing: Evidence-Based Practice Skills*. Oxford, England: Oxford University Press. (See *Frameworks for Critiquing Research Articles*. Available at: http://www.oup.com/uk/orc/bin/9780199563104/01stud ent/chapters/ch07/frameworks/ [Accessed 12 January 2012]).

Websites

An introduction to writing and publishing a systematic review from the Critical Appraisal Skills Programme (CASP). Available at: http://ph.cochrane.org/ sites/ph.cochrane.org/files/uploads/Unit_Eleven.pdf [Accessed 12 April 2012].

Section 2: Writing a Review Article – an introduction to writing a review article for publication. This Section is one of many others related to writing for publication in this guide and it also includes links to other resources that you may find helpful. Available at: http://www.nurseauthoreditor.com/ WritingforPublication2009.pdf [Accessed 12 April 2012].

Chapter 8

Writing for Publication: Turning Assignments into Publishable Works

Mark Hayter

Faculty of Health and Social Care, University of Hull, Hull, UK

Introduction

There must be thousands of excellent essays, assignments, projects and theses gathering dust on the bookshelves of students across the world. Students who have worked hard for a long time are probably pleased to see them put away once they have been submitted, because they think it is the end of the journey. However, this should not be the fate of such work and this chapter looks at how to publish journal papers from academic pieces of work. It takes the standpoint that publication should be the final element in the academic process not the submission to markers/examiners. It intends to be helpful for readers who have either completed or who are about to embark on academic work.

Publication should not be an afterthought. Plan that you will publish your work in some form before you even start your assignment or thesis. If you are undertaking doctoral level study, for example, this should be a core component of your learning agreement with your supervisor and who may also agree to write it with you.

There are numerous ways that you can write up your work, which will enable you to be prepared for later publication. Throughout this chapter you will see how the careful planning of your thesis, dissertation or assignment can pre-empt some of the problems associated with turning academic pieces of work into publishable papers. The chapter starts with some general advice and then looks specifically at the editing and writing challenges associated with different types of papers and how they can be approached.

Writing for Publication in Nursing and Healthcare: Getting It Right, First Edition.
Edited by Karen Holland and Roger Watson.

Get advice on writing your work for publication

Many problems with the road to publication can be avoided by talking to people who are already familiar with it. Colleagues who have adapted academic work for publication can be a valuable resource – talk to them about your ideas. This seems obvious, but can often be hindered by lack of confidence or embarrassment. Try to overcome this because the experiences of others can be vital. If you have a supervisor and have been writing a thesis over a long period, the focus of potential publications should have been discussed early in that supervisory process.

Indeed, a publication, for example the literature review, may already have been undertaken (see Chapter 7). If this has not been discussed yet, raise the topic with your supervisor. For other assignments where this longer process has not happened, seek the help of a more experienced colleague; first, to determine whether the assignment has the potential for a published paper, as not all assignments have, and second, for advice on what type of paper you could write and most importantly the journal you should be aiming to publish your work in.

If this advice has been helpful and you are now clear about what you have to do then you can now plan ahead. If not then you may choose to seek another opinion. However, although more help and advice you get the better, and often thought to be the best way forward, often it can confuse the situation. Choosing who you go to for advice is as important as choosing what you are going to write about from your work; but, be confident; listen to other people but also trust your instinct for a potential paper. For Doctoral level work (a PhD or Professional Doctorate (Prof Doc)), this can also be addressed with examiners who may be well placed to offer advice about potential papers and target journals; take the opportunity to ask. Many experienced examiners will ask this question during the final oral examination or presentation or make recommendations on their examiner's reports, so it is important to note that have thought about it.

Role of supervisors/authorship

As mentioned in Chapter 5, journals have clear guidelines on who qualifies for authorship on a paper and it is important that this is adhered to when publishing academic work. Who is named first on an article is a major issue for many potential authors, in particular if it is in relation to their assignment or study work.

Authorship conventions vary, but it is broadly accepted that if it is their thesis or dissertation that is being used as the foundation of the paper, and they are taking the lead on writing the first draft, the student becomes the first author with the primary supervisor being the second one. Any other authors should then be allocated accordingly if they have had some written input into the article. If they have not had any input but have read the paper and may have offered comments on it, then this must be acknowledged by the author, normally at the end. It is also important to acknowledge in the same way any funding authority that may have funded the student to undertake their course of study.

However authorship is to be decided, it is important that this is discussed by all involved. A further convention in many universities is that, after a specified period, if a student does not publish their work, the supervisor may publish as first author – with the student as second author to ensure authorship convention and ethical practice. These conventions and arrangements vary and students should familiarise themselves with any guidance about this from their own institution.

Activity 1

Find out the convention and requirements of your programme of study for writing articles as it applies in your university/college. Discuss this with your academic supervisor and plan for future publications.

What type of publication?

How and where you publish your academic work depends, among other things, on the type of work written or produced. Chapter 2 provides some advice on targeting journals, but for academic assignments the following issues are identified. Academic pieces of work take many forms but can broadly be summarised into the following four categories:

(1) Essays that focus on a particular clinical or professional issue, discuss the literature (but that do not systematically search the literature; See Chapter 7) and comment on the implications for practice.
(2) Concept analysis or theoretical papers – focusing on a particular aspect of your study background.
(3) Literature reviews, meta-analysis or meta-ethnography.
(4) Research studies that include background and context of the research, together with the research design, data analysis and findings, discussion and recommendations.

Essays

Structured essays are the most common type of assignment in academic programmes of study but are also the most difficult academic pieces of work to get published. Obviously, it depends on what it has been written for and also the academic level it is meant to be aimed for. It is also important to recognise that because a tutor has marked the assignment and given feedback that '*this is an excellent piece of work and you should consider getting it published*', it can actually then be turned into an actual article for publication. This is mainly due to the fact that it has been written for a completely different purpose and most of the time to strict and structured guidelines.

However some postgraduate programmes now have 'essay' assignments, which require students to write this in the form of an article for publication, following specific journal guidelines and word limitations. This of course offers the student an added advantage of having already mapped out an article for a specific journal.

For others who have not undertaken this type of essay the target journal is important, as is the 'message' of what you wish to convey (see Chapter 5). It is very unlikely that a high-impact international peer-review journal will publish a paper that has begun its journey as an essay. That is not to say it is impossible depending on the type of essay it is and also whether it can be added to in terms of further literature and evidence; that is, it can be used as the foundation for a different level of academic rigour and scholarship.

The immediate target journal (again depending on the message to be conveyed and the target readership) could be a regional or national level journal, which may or may not be linked to professional practice. Even then work will be required to convert an essay into an article. The positive aspect of an essay is that it will most probably have a structure of an introduction or background, aims to be achieved, a 'middle' section where the literature will have been evidenced and 'an end' where discussion will have been undertaken along with recommendations for practice and or future research.

Regardless of what type of assignment or assessed work we are starting with, it is important to follow some of the steps highlighted in Chapters 5 and 2. Initially think about what the focus of the article should be – if the essay or assignment has been about a clinical evidence-based case study, then a journal that focuses on education will not be suitable for the paper. An initial Internet search, inserting topic titles such as sexual health journal or mental health practice journal will often suffice. This will highlight a number of journals.

Activity 2

Try searching for journals as stated: sexual health journal and mental health practice journal. What type of journals did you find and how many would be suitable for a publication from a student assignment?

In a quick search via Google the following journals were found:

Sexual Health Journals:

Sexual Health (CSIRO Publishing)
International Journal of Sexual Health (Taylor Francis On-line)
Sexually Transmitted Infections (BMJ Journals)
Perspectives on Sexual and Reproductive Health (Wiley-Blackwell Publications)

Mental Health Journals:

Mental Health Practice Magazine (RCN Publishing)

The Journal of Mental Health Training, Education, and Practice (Mental Health in Higher Education - Higher Education Academy)

International Journal of Mental Health Nursing (Wiley-Blackwell Publications)

Journal of Rural Mental Health (Open Journal Systems)

Once you have found one or two journals that you think may be suitable for your essay style paper, look at a selection of them and think how your assignment could be adapted. One area that you will need to think about for practice-focused journals and articles is that the paper will need to be clear about the implications for practice, policy or service provision - if these issues are not explicit in your assignment then this will require attention in your revision of it for publication.

If the essay addresses a local issue then can this be expanded to encompass wider, national concerns? Even national and regional professional journals will expect this and will be unlikely to publish papers that just address a local issue, unless it can be used as a case study example. A positive note is that word counts for professional journals may be close to the word counts of academic essays and editing out lots of material may not be required.

And finally for papers derived from essays; an essay, as noted previously, that is well written and planned in the first place - has a clear introduction, logically structured (for adaptation into sections if a journal requires this), makes clear points about the implications for practice and has a clear, concise conclusion - will be all the easier to adapt for publication.

Concept analysis or theoretical papers

These types of assignments have more potential for international publications, mainly because of the need to ensure that the content base arises from all types of evidence. These papers usually arise from postgraduate work, but some undergraduate dissertations can also produce material worthy of being considered for translation into published paper. It is important that you discuss this with either your supervisor or another tutor that has published articles in various journals or who may even be a journal editor. Some organisations will also have writing for publication workshops to help new authors get their work published, and where students or staff are expected to bring draft work or assignments with them to the sessions.

It is worth reading Chapters 2 and 5 for considering how to approach writing for this kind of article, but whatever you decide to write about or write for please remember it is important to consider the international reader (Holland, 2005). Holland (2005) makes this point in relation to medical students writing for publication, and it equally applies to other healthcare professional students:

> It is interesting to note that general advice to potential authors in studentBMJ *(an international magazine for medical students) offers the following note of advice:*
>
> Remember that the studentBMJ *(www.student.BMJ.com) has a broad international readership, so try, as far as possible, to keep your articles internationally relevant and keep the language as simple as possible (you are writing to communicate a message, not to show off how many long words you know).*
>
> *(Holland, 2005, p. 1)*

Literature reviews and systematic reviews

As with concept analysis, many leading international journals publish well-written and well-conducted reviews of the literature. The important words here being 'well-written and well-conducted'. Although not expecting a full systematic review, most journals will not accept a literature review paper without a substantial methodology section that outlines a rigorous search strategy. Again, it is important to recall who the readership is and what message you are trying to convey, together with remembering that your article is being developed from an assignment or a chapter in a thesis or postgraduate dissertation. It goes without saying that it is expected that any review of literature should already be at a level where it can be considered for translation to an article.

At a minimum, databases, search terms, dates and inclusion/exclusion criteria should be outlined and also a clear account of the search results. To this effect, a diagram or table can be worth hundreds of words and editors will be looking particularly for the use of a flow chart, such as the PRISMA one illustrated here (Figure 8.1).

Following the description of a search strategy and results, the methods section should also contain a description of how the literature was appraised and again, a table that comprises a 'matrix' type model is helpful – a table breaking down the research papers into their component parts for appraisal (Table 8.1).

There is also a growing recognition in leading journals that something 'more' may be required than a thorough and rigorous review of the literature. There is a trend towards authors being encouraged to conduct meta-analysis of quantitative research papers or a meta-synthesis/ethnography of qualitative studies.

This is clearly a fact to be considered when embarking on an academic piece of work – and may be precluded by assessment guidelines – but, if students have a choice it could be a positive one to make with regard to future publication potential. This book is not about these methods, therefore

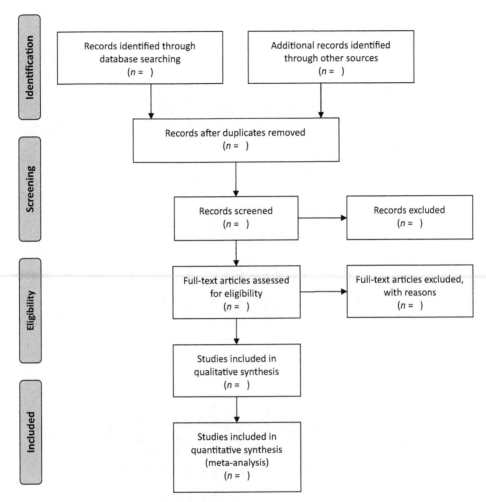

Figure 8.1 PRISMA 2009 flow diagram. (From Moher, D., Liberati, A., Tetzlaff, J., Altman, D.G. & The PRISMA Group (2009) *Preferred Reporting Items for Systematic Reviews and Meta-Analyses: the PRISMA Statement. PLoS Medicine* 6(6), e1000097. doi:10.1371/journal.pmed1000097. For more information, visit www.prisma-statement.org.)

a detailed account of these approaches will not be provided (see Further reading).

It should be noted also that a meta-analysis (i.e. a systematic review and analysis of 'quantitative studies' and their data) requires a great deal of statistical skill and would normally be carried out by experienced researchers who may or may not be undertaking further study, such as a PhD by publication, for example. On the other hand, a meta-synthesis/ethnography (see Campbell et al. (2003) – the analysis of qualitative studies) could be written for publication in similar circumstances (see Atkins et al., 2008).

Table 8.1 Empirical research matrix.

Author and date	Design	Aims	Sample type and size	Data collection	Ethics	Summary of findings	Limitations	Discussion	Themes
Title of paper	Qualitative	To investigate whether physicians discussed issues surrounding the end of life with patient and/or their relatives.	A random sample of 300 physicians was drawn from the professional register of specialities frequently involved in the end of life.	A questionnaire with structured questions was posted to practising physicians in seven countries: (1) Australia (2) Belgium (3) Denmark (4) Italy (5) the Netherlands (6) Sweden (7) Switzerland	None discussed	Significant cross-national differences were identified in this study, as communication is typical of many traditionally Catholic countries.	Response rates were not high. Physicians were not asked to consider a specific diagnostic category when responding to the communication questions.	The majority of physicians in most of the participating countries except Italy discuss issues related to the end of life with their patients, but not always with relatives.	Patient wishes Patient understanding Withdrawing treatment

Research studies

Longer pieces of academic work such as empirical research studies have the most potential for publication. They are likely to have been conducted using recognised research methods and have 'new' findings to present.

In a PhD there may be an opportunity for several linked papers – consider this if you have clearly distinctive and separate issues/concepts to discuss. Think about the potential for a theoretical paper, a clinically focused paper and a methodological paper also. As long as separate papers clearly refer to each other then this type of approach is acceptable. An issue to avoid is the accusation of 'salami slicing' (Norman and Griffiths, 2008) – where very similar papers on closely related topics are published from one piece of research with little to distinguish them apart. If there are different aspects of the data to be presented, for example data related to patients and data related to professionals, think about two linked papers in one journal (Part 1 and Part 2). Journals will consider this type of linked papers and editors can be contacted prior to submission if necessary to check if this is acceptable. It must be clear, however, that a though the articles may be linked, they should be viewed as single separate articles but cross-referenced to each other, as they normally present different aspects of a study or development. Your supervisor or well-published colleague would be able to advise you on this approach.

Another consideration is that a longer paper that contains several elements may be more valuable than shorter and separate, fragmented papers. Of course, this depends on the word limits of various journals, with a journal such as *Journal of Advanced Nursing* having a 5000-word limit but *Sociology of Health & Illness* having 8000 words. Others require less words and the danger is that submitting a paper that is too long may well be a rejection or at best returned to you for further editing and then re-submission. This is time wasting and can be discouraging. During your studies you will be learning how to make maximum use of word limits and it is best that this practice is maintained when you are writing for publication as well as your thesis, dissertation or essays.

The longer paper may allow you however to discuss an issue thoroughly and present substantial findings, especially important when writing qualitative research requiring narrative examples. The less positive aspect is that they are usually considerably longer than the word limit of journals and substantial editing is required. The following sections of this chapter look at this process in detail.

Editing research dissertations and theses for publication

This can be one of the most difficult tasks both during the course of your study and after completion. Normally undergraduate dissertations can be anything up to 10,000 words and a Doctoral study (PhD) could be between 80,000 and 100,000 words! This can make the task of producing a 5000–6000 word paper look daunting. Many authors are unable to achieve editing their work for publication, seeing it as too much of a challenge after already having written so many words.

The following are some key areas involved in the writing of an article from a large research study and the editing process, and is based on the assumption that a peer-review international journal where you have chosen to publish your work will require a paper length of 5000–6000 words (you are lucky to get more!) and, similar to Chapter 5, the suggested and approximate breakdown of this research study article could be as follows:

- Introduction/background or literature review *1000–1500 words.*
- Methods (all elements of the research process) *750–1000 words.*
- Results/findings *1000–2000 words* (although, it will vary dependant on the nature of the data. It could be considerably less for quantitative data that judiciously uses tables.).
- Discussion *1500–2500 words.*
- Conclusion/implications for practice *500–750 words* (some journals ask for more here).

This is a rough guide only, because you may decide that the focus of the publication will be on the findings and discussion, and the methodology and research design will be discussed in more detail in another paper, especially if it is innovative and has led to original new ideas and practice.

As discussed in Chapter 2, checking the journal guidelines for authors is an essential step once a journal has been selected. Obtain a sample paper (recently published, as journal guidelines can change) that closely matches your type of work – this will give you a good sense of what type of material is provided in each of the sections of the paper (and, importantly – what is not) and the level of detail required in sections, such as data collection, sampling, discussion, etc. At this point it could be that the type of journal style may not reflect your assignment/thesis or your ideas for your paper. Do not try to force your work to fit – it may be more productive to review your choice of journal at this stage.

Begin to think that you will have to lose many of your words. This sounds obvious, but your task will involve a lot more than simply reducing a few paragraphs. To focus on what you have to do you need to prepare to remove what you might think is some of your best writing – which it may be – but that was for your academic supervisor or examiner, not a reader in a journal. Developing the ability to be ruthless with your own work is hard, but essential for turning a long academic assignment into a publication. Also, be clear from the start that it will not purely be an editing task that involves reducing a word count. It will certainly involve this, but you will probably have to re-write and add extra material and re-structure your current work. This is particularly important with regard to any new evidence that has been discovered since you wrote your final piece of work; and also, the readership or audience is different. Note again that it is important to consider the international reader of the journal. This cannot be done hastily and editors do not like to receive quickly edited theses to consider, sometimes even with the original section numbering, and this will be likely to result in early rejection of the submitted work even before review.

If you are new to writing articles get some help. Ideally from your supervisor who, acting as a co-author, will have less of an emotional attachment to the work and may also be experienced in this type of editing. If this is not possible, seek out the advice of a more experienced colleague on the type of material you can safely remove.

If they have time they may offer to help with this editing, after you have tried it yourself. The key issue that one must return to again and again is the question of who is the article aimed at and what messages are needed to be considered in the writing process. It is not just about cutting sections here and there, you must have a cohesive wholeness to the paper.

This is equally so for translating research reports you may have written for a funding body into an article for publication. Give your peer reviewer permission to be hard with their editing – material can always be replaced again if need be.

> ### Tip 1
>
> Make sure you keep a master copy of the assignment/thesis safely. Create separate files for all the papers being developed from your work. In fact it may be prudent as well to keep copies in a separate place, such as a USB data stick. This is because the editing process – in addition to removing material – often involves a review and a decision to reinstate material that you may have deleted. Editing is like writing in that you add and take away – but editing often works the other way round.

Introduction and background/literature review

A crucial first step is to look at your target journal and how they structure this section of the paper (read the author guidelines again). Secondly, these sections of the thesis will probably be very long, may actually include three or four chapters and will need reducing to about 1000–1500 words. Begin with shortening your introduction to give a good idea of the focus and importance of the study. Keep it brief, for example:

Married couples who fail to bear children are commonly stigmatized (Donkor and Sandal, 2007) or disqualified from 'full' social acceptance (Dyer et al., 2002). It has also been reported that childlessness could lead to marital dissatisfaction (Lee and Sun, 2000; Dyer et al., 2002). Understanding how sub-fertility is experienced can be valuable for practitioners involved in numerous areas of family nursing (Callister, 1995). However, there is little literature that explores this topic from a Chinese cultural perspective, particularly among Hong Kong Chinese, a gap this qualitative paper is designed to address.

The above example is just 91 words long but tells the reader all they need to know in an introduction. This is also good practice for when you return to write the abstract for the paper, which has to include all aspects of your study, and from which individuals searching the databases will be able determine what the paper is all about.

Tip 2

Do not forget to state the aims of the paper itself, normally after this section. The reader needs to know what this is, not just what the aims of the actual study being reported is.

The introduction is usually followed by some sort of literature review or background and in many studies this can extend over two or three chapters. If the paper being written, however, is itself a systematically conducted review of the literature, then it is these chapters that will be the core ones to be edited. Either situation will mean a significant editing task.

It is important that, when editing this section, the following principles are applied. *First*, make sure that the key literature is included. *Second*, look at the dates of literature in your review – try to be more contemporary (while not removing seminal or influential historical references). *Third*, make sure that any editing done does not lose the international importance of the context of the study. This is where many papers are weak, possibly due to editing, in that they concentrate too much on local/national literature and fail to put the study in an international context. This could be, of course, a limitation of the original section in the thesis. If this is the case, then prior to publication submission more work should be undertaken in rectifying this section to add international literature but also ensuring that any local/national issues are briefly explained for the international reader (see Chapters 2 and 5).

The methods section

This section in a journal's author guidelines is more often than not called the methods section, but is in fact the content expected in it, including all the research design elements. This aspect of your thesis will be likely to require a substantial reduction in words. Journal styles differ but most nursing journals that publish research articles require a description of the aim of the study or research question, the methodology, the methods, sampling, ethical issues, participants, data collection and data analysis – the latter often with a section on rigour or trustworthiness depending on the research approach adopted. This description of the methods will usually be separated into explicit subsections under a generic 'methodology' or 'method' heading.

When editing these sections of your thesis, as with the background, think of what is essential to give a clear description of the study. Starting with the methodology, there may be considerable narrative in a thesis about this. A journal editor will not be interested in a long debate in a thesis about the relative merits of quantitative versus qualitative research, or of a detailed comparison of different approaches within the chosen genre. A few sentences will often suffice to address this, for example, the following was edited from a 2000 words methodological debate in a thesis:

> Informed by the aim, a qualitative, exploratory method utilising a phenomenological approach was used. Phenomenology focuses on individual interpretations of lived experiences and the ways in which they are expressed (Parahoo, 1997). Phenomenology is a qualitative, inductive methodology, designed to elicit participant's perceived experiences, seeking to attribute meanings to participant's narratives and present an overall picture of the phenomenon under investigation.
>
> (Omery, 1983; Munhall and Olier, 1986)

Note that the above example clearly draws relevance to the research question. This is really all that may be required here.

Data collection methods and analysis

How data were collected and analysed is of course dependent on the methodology and methods used, and terminology used will therefore differ. The important issues to put in this section(s) are: the technique of sampling used and its congruence with the methodology, and the practical ways it was achieved. The nature and number of participants is also essential here. This may be in a brief narrative, for example:

> All of the participants were born in, and had lived in, Hong Kong all their lives. The women were 36–44 years old, and the men were 36–45 years old. They had been married between 8 and 22 years. Among the four interviewed couples, one couple had been educated to primary school level (occupations were sales lady and taxi-driver), two couples had completed secondary school (all had white collar positions), and another couple both had university education (both professionals).

It can also be illustrated as in Table 8.2.

The most important issue to remember here is to ensure accuracy and congruence of the methodology and methods used in the thesis.

Table 8.2 (a) Participant demographics; (b) participant information.

(a) Item	Number	Percentage
Gender		
Male	6	66.7
Female	3	33.3
Age		
30~39 yr	1	11.1
40~49 yr	4	44.5
50~59 yr	3	33.3
60~69 yr	1	11.1
Married status		
Married	7	77.8
Single	2	22.2
Employment status		
Employed	8	88.9
Unemployed	1	11.1
Myasthenia gravis type		
Generalised type	6	66.7
Ocular type	3	33.3

(b) Name (anonymous)	Age	Gender	Married status	Employment	Type of MG	Voluntary
Chih	64	M	Married	Employed	Generalised	Yes
Han	55	M	Married	Employed	Ocular	No
Hsiung	45	F	Single	Employed	Generalised	Yes
Hsun	46	M	Married	Employed	Generalised	Yes
Jia	42	F	Married	Unemployed	Generalised	Yes
Waie	36	M	Single	Employed	Generalised	Yes
Wen	50	M	Married	Employed	Generalised	Yes
Yauw	43	M	Married	Employed	Ocular	No
Ying	53	F	Married	Retired	Generalised	Yes

Ethical considerations

This is an essential section for all journals that publish research articles. Any research article that does not report that the required ethical permission to conduct the study has been obtained will not be considered by editors. This cannot be undertaken retrospectively. If you want to publish the findings from a research study then it is assumed that during the conduct of your thesis this had been obtained. Editors will expect to see a clear statement on this at the start of this section, for example:

This study was approved by the (name the institution here) Research Ethics Committee on the (date here).

Some studies however will report that this Ethics Committee permission was granted by both an academic institution and an external organisation such as the National Health Service in the UK.

Following this statement, a brief discussion of the steps to be taken to address the ethical dimensions of the study can be undertaken. It is likely that a Master's or Doctoral dissertation/thesis will have a long section on these issues, maybe with an associated discussion of ethical theory/principles or frameworks. Unless absolutely necessary, this kind of theoretical debate does not need to be included in an article for publication that is reporting on the whole study. Keep only to the key principles in this section: how were participants informed about the study and how was informed consent achieved, confidentiality assured and were subjects informed that they could leave the study without pressure? For research projects that involve sensitive issues, the matter of how potential distress among participants was handled will also require a mention.

Data collection methods

As with the methodology, brevity is needed. A thesis/dissertation may concern extensive debate about alternative data collection methods. It may be wise to pre-empt reviewer questions on this with a brief mention of, why, for example, interviews were chosen over focus groups, but prolonged debate that includes methods not even used in the paper are not required, neither is an extensive discussion about the development of any instruments used. With qualitative research interviews, what type of interviews and (briefly) why this was important need to be included, and if interview schedules were used give example questions. This can be also be written in the form of a table – another word saving strategy.

Data analysis

Again, this section should include the important issues only. What tests were used for example and why (ensuring congruence with methodology is important), and a brief but clear explanation of the analysis procedures. To describe the analysis can a table be used? This helps with the word count as tables and figures are not included in this word count by most journals. Even in qualitative

Table 8.3 Extract from an observed consultation between nurse and patient (clinic A).

Extract from consultation 6 (clinic A)	Open codes
Nurse: What we suggest you do is start your pill from whatever date your period starts and from then on you are sort of protected.	*Instructions on use* *Protection from pregnancy*
Woman: The last day...?	*Women questioning*
Nurse: No, the first day of your period, so whatever day of the week that is, and you carry on for all your 21 pills. We suggest you take it at the same time every day, it doesn't matter what time of day it is, whatever suits your lifestyle. It's best if you get up at the same time in the morning and are able to remember to take it with your first cup of coffee at breakfast.	*Awareness of menstruation* *Being aware of time* *Instruction in use* *Fitting into lifestyle*
Woman: Yes.	*Affirming understanding*
Nurse: What we suggest you do is take it at the same time everyday within a few hours.	*Awareness of time* *Instructions on use*
Woman: I tend to do that.	*Confirming compliance*
Nurse: That's great. This is the leaflet we will be giving you to go through. The pill is over 99% effective, but that depends on how well you take it, if you forget to take it and go messing around with the times, then it is not so effective.	*Giving written information* *Contraceptive% efficacy* *Danger of non-compliance* *Interference with contraception*

papers – a table can be a useful way of illustrating an example of how thematic coding was achieved (and save a large number of words). Table 8.3 is an example of this in practice and illustrates coding in grounded theory.

Presenting the findings

It is here that quantitative researchers have a distinct advantage. Most statistical data can be presented in tables with relatively little accompanying narrative. Existing tables and figures from a thesis can probably be used without any adaptation. However, think carefully about the number of tables, as journals not only have restricted word limits but they also have what are known as 'page budgets' (see Chapter 10), that is each volume of a journal has allocated number of pages for printing articles. If an article you submit has many tables but the required number of words, your paper may be rejected or you may be asked to reduce the number. Many authors may not be aware of these additional considerations.

The amount of data presented here needs to address the aims of the paper. If too much data is being presented it may mean the discussion section cannot handle all the issues from the data. In this event it may be worth re-visiting the potential for linked papers as already discussed earlier.

It is actually the qualitative researcher who has the greatest task when attempting to choose data and findings from their research. The data in a qualitative research thesis is often extensive. This is necessary to demonstrate rigour and to satisfy the requirements of examiners/markers that you have actually collected the data and analysed it. In a PhD/MPhil this maybe 10,000-15,000 words. In a journal paper you will not have the luxury of being able to present your qualitative data extensively – it must be edited down. This is not easy, but is one of the most important editing steps. This must also be done while keeping the key findings intact and supporting your findings with the data. Qualitative data are usually presented by thematic sections that consist of a continuous, linking narrative interspersed with extracts from the data to support this narrative. It is a matter of judgement how to reduce this work (often from the longest section of a thesis) to a section of about 2000 words, but the following will help:

Tip 3

(1) Make sure you report all your themes. This is not a time to revise your initial analysis. If they were important before they are important now.

(2) Look carefully at the data extracts. If two are used to support one point in your narrative can one be removed?

(3) Are minor points in your narrative supported by too much data – can any be lost without detriment to your message?

(4) Make sure that your data remains representative of the participants. Reviewers of papers will look to make sure that authors have not over-relied on just a few participants. This is a common failing when qualitative data is edited. Check for this.

(5) Finally read through the written sections – do they repeat what the data is saying – are there any areas where the data can be made to speak for itself. The narrative should be edited as well as the data – try to tell the story as succinctly as possible.

Rigour

Many of the leading journals ask for specific information on the techniques that have been used to ensure the findings are trustworthy or reliable. Clearly, this should have been part of the original study. If a long section of this has been written this should be edited to about 200 words at most. Clear reference to the literature on rigour should start this section, followed by the specific techniques used to ensure it.

Discussion section

This is one of the most important sections of any publication and the require-ments for a thesis are likely to mean that this section will require major editing and the addition of new material. As mentioned earlier, thinking about future publication can help these sections of the thesis to be written in a way to reduce the editing task later but of course this must not take precedence over what is required for your thesis to be complete, and in fact editing your final draft of a thesis will already have helped your skills in doing this.

Keep methodological discussion separate from any narrative that places the findings in context with the associated literature. This latter issue is very important in an article, as it demonstrates not only understanding of their relationship but also that the findings are clearly evidence based.

Write separate sections for the implications for practice and policy, some journals may specify that an article should include this for publication in that journal (check the guidelines again). One section may address local is-sues, whereas a separate section looks at wider international policy/practice relevance.

For many international journals the inclusion of a discussion of the inter-national relevance of the study is an essential requirement. Many papers are rejected because this aspect is weak or not present, especially if the author guidelines make this very clear. This is not the same as making the actual article understandable for the international readership. It must be noted that not all research reported in articles can be relevant in other countries, but may offer solutions to similar situations or dilemmas.

This disappointment can be avoided by realistically targeting the paper to a specific journal (as discussed earlier) or by ensuring that this section has noted a possible international relevance. If this element is not in the original academic work then it will need to be added. This is where the extra work comes in – here the emphasis moves from editing and reducing words to actually adding new material.

The important aspect here is to compare and contrast the findings of your study with the international literature, which should already have been con-sidered in your thesis. A publishable paper will identify and discuss how and why your paper adds to the literature by providing a different insight (maybe cultural or geographical) to the empirical understanding of a topic and clearly set out the implications of this new understanding for further research and practice. Papers that merely reinforce the findings of other studies in the same field or do not attempt to critically review these are not as sought after by editors who may have to choose to accept one article to publish out of every ten submitted.

Essential to this discussion section is, however, the 'new' knowledge or con-tribution that your research makes to the wider scholarship of the discipline and that in your thesis may have been attributed to the notion of 'originality'. This may have been part of the original project and as such any paper that expand or develop internationally existing theoretical understanding is valued not only by journal editors but also by other researchers worldwide. This will also add to the use of your article by others who will cite your work in theirs and increase both your citation counts as well as the journal's.

Limitations

Many leading journals require authors to describe the limitations of their work, especially if it is a research study. This section is often hastily written but it is important to state if there were limitations that could have affected that actual findings of the research and therefore any recommendations reported. However, most Doctoral studies will have weaknesses of one kind or another and honesty is required. A good suggestion here for authors is to turn limitations into positives by linking them to the need for further research, as the following extract illustrates:

This study has a number of limitations but these also provide opportunities for further research in this area. Firstly, participants in the study were only followed up for one week. Given that complications of a stoma may arise following discharge from the hospital future studies with one, six and twelve month follow-ups might prove informative. Secondly, participants were recruited from only one medical centre and the results from multi-centre trial would be more generalisable. Thirdly, outcome indicators only used self-reported data making it somewhat difficult to ascertain the level of correlation between actual stoma self-care and self-reported behaviours. Consequently, further research is recommended, utilizing measures that involve directly observed stoma self-care behaviour to compare with the findings of this study.

Article conclusion and recommendations for practice

This will require a short paragraph only, and it is not the place to recommence discussion and introduction of new material. It should stick to the key points and implications of the study. Some journals ask for a section on the relevance to practice as part of a conclusion. The conclusion will bring together your own assessment of the research conducted and reported in your article, and the final task you will need to undertake in a similar way is to now write the abstract.

The article abstract

The abstract you are required to write should encapsulate your whole research study if it is to be of value to other researchers in their searching of databases as well as demonstrating that you can present your work in a clear and concise way. An abstract is an essential requirement of a research article, although some journals who accept other types of papers may not require this. Again, please refer to the author guidance on this (see Chapters 2 and 5 for further information on abstracts and submission of articles).

See examples of abstracts in Boxes 8.1 and 8.2.

Box 8.1 Abstract 1 (structured guidelines and word limits)

Bailey, C., Murphy, R. & Porrock, D. (2011) Professional tears: developing emotional intelligence around death and dying in emergency work. *Journal of Clinical Nursing*, 20(23-24), 3364-3372

Abstract

Key words
- Accident and emergency
- Emergency department
- Emotional aspects
- End-of-life care
- Nurse–patient relationship
- Nursing care

Aims and objectives: This paper explores how emergency nurses manage the emotional impact of death and dying in emergency work and presents a model for developing expertise in end-of-life care delivery.

Background: Care of the dying, the deceased and the bereaved is largely conducted by nurses, and nowhere is this more demanding than at the front door of the hospital, the Emergency Department. While some nurses find end-of-life care a rewarding aspect of their role, others avoid opportunities to develop a relationship with the dying and bereaved because of the intense and exhausting nature of the associated emotional labour.

Design: Qualitative study using unstructured observations of practice and semi-structured interviews.

Methods: Observation was conducted in a large Emergency Department over 12 months. We also conducted 28 in-depth interviews with emergency staff, patients with terminal illnesses and their relatives.

Results: Emergency nurses develop expertise in end-of-life care giving by progressing through three stages of development: (1) investment of the self in the nurse–patient relationship, (2) management of emotional labour and (3) development of emotional intelligence. Barriers that prevent the transition to expertise contribute to occupational stress and can lead to burnout and withdrawal from practice.

Conclusions: Despite the emotional impact of emergency deaths, nurses who invest their therapeutic self into the nurse–patient relationship are able to manage the emotional labour of caring for the dying and their relatives through the development of emotional intelligence. They find reward in end-of-life care that ultimately creates a more positive experience for patients and their relatives.

Relevance to clinical practice: The emergency nurse caring for the dying patient is placed in a unique and privileged position to make a considerable impact on the care of the patient and the experience for their family. This model can build awareness in managing the emotive aspects involved in care delivery and develop fundamental skills of nursing patients near the end of life.

Box 8.2   Abstract (word limit guidelines only)

Pickles, D., King, L. & Belan, I. (2011) Undergraduate nursing students' attitudes towards caring for people with HIV/AIDS. *Nurse Education Today,* 32(1), 15-20.

Summary

The aim of this quantitative study was to determine the attitudes of Australian nursing students towards caring for people with HIV/AIDS. This research study was conducted among second year undergraduate nursing students at a university in South Australia, during August 2007. The survey tool consisted of six demographic questions and the AIDS Attitude Scale. This questionnaire was completed by 396 students, giving a response rate of 94.7%. The vast majority (95.7%) of students participating in this study demonstrated very positive attitudes towards caring for people with HIV/AIDS and only 4.3% demonstrated negative attitudes. No statistically significant differences were found in attitude score based on participants' age, gender, previous HIV/AIDS education, previous nursing experience or previous experience of caring for someone with HIV/AIDS. A statistically significant difference in AIDS attitude score was found in relation to participants' country/region of citizenship, with nursing students from China, East Asia, South East Asia and Central Asia and Middle East having more negative attitudes than students from other countries/regions. As an increasing number of nursing students have been recruited to Australia from these countries/regions, nurse educators need to be aware of such differences when planning and delivering HIV/AIDS educational programs in tertiary institutions.

Key words: Nursing education, Nursing students, HIV/AIDS, Attitudes, Research

Conclusion

This chapter has described how to develop an article for publication from academic pieces of work, in particular a research thesis. It provides a range of advice and issues to consider in undertaking this important contribution to scholarship and the evidence base of a discipline. However, it is important that author guidelines are read carefully before any submission is made to a journal, whatever type of article you wish to write and publish from any academic work. It must be stressed that this chapter is also not a replacement for the advice and help of more experienced colleagues especially those with writing and editing experience.

Writing an article or articles for publication should be a part of any post-graduate or doctoral student's academic agreement and it is hoped that the guidance offered in this chapter together with that in other relevant chapters will enable you to at least have the confidence to attempt to write up the outcome of your hard work into an accepted publication.

References

Atkins, S., Lewin, S., Smith, H., Engel, M., Fretheim, A. & Volmink, J. (2008) Conducting a meta-ethnography of qualitative research: lessons learnt. *BMC Medical Research Methodology*, 8, 21.

Campbell, R., Pound, P., Pope, C., Britten, N., Pill, R., Morgan, M. & Donovan, J. (2003) Evaluating metaethnography: a synthesis of qualitative research on lay experiences of diabetes and diabetes care. *Social Science and Medicine*, 56(4), 671-684.

Holland, K. (2005) Writing for an international readership. *Nurse Education in Practice*, 5, 1-2.

Munhall, P.L. & Oiler, C.J. (1986) *Nursing Research: A Qualitative Perspective*. Norwalk, CT: Appleton-Century-Crofts.

Norman, I. & Griffiths, P. (2008) Duplicate publication and 'salami slicing': ethical issues and practical solutions. *International Journal of Nursing Studies*, 45(9), 1257-1260.

Omery, A. (1983) Phenomenology: a method for nursing research. *Advances in Nursing Science*, 5(2), 49-63.

Further reading

Epstein, D., Kenway, J. & Boden, R. (2005) *Writing for Publication*. London: Sage Publications.

Hartley, J. (2008) *Academic Writing and Publishing – A Practical Handbook*. Abingdon: Routledge.

Woods, P. (2005) *Successful Writing for Qualitative Researchers*. Abingdon: Routledge.

Chapter 9

Writing for Publication: Turning the Conference Paper into Publishable Work

Tracy Levett-Jones and Teresa Stone

School of Nursing and Midwifery, Faculty of Health, University of Newcastle, Callaghan, NSW, Australia

> *Good writing is like a windowpane*
> *George Orwell*

Introduction

To a large extent nursing has evolved as an oral tradition where insights, learned experiences and knowledge are transmitted to others through both informal means (e.g. clinical conversations) and more formal approaches such as in-services, seminars and conferences. For this reason many nurses feel more confident presenting at conferences than they do writing for publication. The primary purpose of a conference paper is knowledge dissemination; however, unless presented as a keynote presentation or plenary session, the audience is often relatively small and the conference paper is of benefit only to the people who attend the session. The opportunity to reach a much wider number of people over an extended period is afforded when one's conference paper is transformed into a published paper. This is not as challenging as it might sound and in this chapter we share with you some strategies that will make this both possible and enjoyable.

The chapter begins by discussing some of the benefits of turning a conference paper into a publication; we then confront some of the challenges associated with doing this. Nurses and other health professionals often relate to examples, stories and shared experiences; for this reason, we provide some of our own examples of transforming conference papers into publications and what we have learnt along the way. We conclude with a *Checklist for Success* (see Table 9.1); it provides a relatively simple process for creating conference papers and published works concurrently.

Writing for Publication in Nursing and Healthcare: Getting It Right, First Edition.
Edited by Karen Holland and Roger Watson.
© 2012 John Wiley & Sons, Ltd. Published 2012 by John Wiley & Sons, Ltd.

Table 9.1 Checklist for success.

Title of presentation: Title of manuscript: Authors: Conference abstract submission date: Date of conference: Planned date for submission of manuscript:	√	Comments
I have checked the conference abstract requirements.		
I have checked the author guidelines for the journal.		
My co-authors and I have agreed on our contributions to the presentation and manuscript. This agreement has been documented.		
The timeline for the preparation of the conference presentation and submission of manuscript has been prepared.		
I have a plan to complete the final draft of the conference abstract *at least one month prior* to the due date to enable peer review.		
The presentation/manuscript is supported by relevant and current literature.		
The presentation/manuscript is referenced according to journal guidelines.		
References are organised so they can easily be retrieved.		
I have a system for filing, backing up and dating all drafts.		
Feedback from peers has been taken into account in the development of the presentation and manuscript.		
The conference paper has been developed according to guidelines in Chapter 3.		
Questions and feedback from the conference audience have been considered in finalising the journal manuscript.		
The manuscript has been developed according to guidelines in Chapter 5.		
Issues related to ethics, permissions, competing interests and acknowledgments have been addressed and dealt with appropriately.		

The benefits of turning a conference paper into a published work

Professional and scholarly conferences provide a valuable but somewhat limited opportunity to exchange knowledge. However, when the conference paper is turned into a publication we become part of a community of scholarship and we contribute to the ongoing advancement of nursing practice and knowledge (Stone et al., 2010). The art of writing enables us to present our thoughts, findings and arguments on a given subject, whether it be a clinical, educational or research project (Stone et al., 2010). There is an emerging professional expectation for health professionals to publish findings from research and innovative practice development initiatives (Taylor et al., 2005; Murray and Newton, 2008). Some even suggest that there is an obligation to publish (Winslow et al., 1996, 2008), and that it may be unethical not to do so (Savitz, 2000).

The development of a publishable work from a conference paper can increase research productivity (Lee and Boud, 2003), enhance self-esteem (Baldwin and Chandler, 2002), promote clinical improvement (Dixon, 2001) and contribute to a body of professional knowledge. Although this takes time and commitment there are many advantages. Much of the work for the paper has already been completed during the process of preparing the conference presentation: the literature will have been reviewed, the project designed, implemented and evaluated and a coherent presentation created. When you develop the presentation and the paper concurrently, the benefits are increased and the workload reduced.

Conferences are an excellent opportunity to meet journal editors. Editors often attend academic conferences to find out what is happening in the areas they publish in. It is worthwhile introducing yourself and discussing whether your work aligns with their journal's aims and scope (VanEvery, 2011). Conference presentations also provide a wonderful opportunity to share knowledge and experiences in a way that allows for immediate interaction and feedback from the audience through comments and questions. Critical feedback is valuable and can be used to gauge the interest in the topic and strengthen your paper before submitting it for publication. If you have presented at a conference and someone has asked, 'Have you published that?', you know that you have generated interest in a topic that may be relevant to other nurses and or health professionals. Apart from feeling pleased and proud that your work has made an impact, you should consider whether to take the next step into the world of scholarly pursuits. Questions to consider at this stage include:

- Does your work add to and extend upon the work of others? Is it novel, innovative, interesting and does it break new ground? The best way to test this out is, of course, to search the published literature. Unless your work contributes significantly to what is already known, it may not be accepted for publication.
- To whom and how broadly is your work of interest? Most international journals seek papers of international relevance. If your work is a small localised study then it may be better to consider a local journal or a publication for an interest group.

- Who could you work with in writing the paper? Academic or research colleagues who can support and guide you through the publication process will make the journey easier and more enjoyable.

Despite the benefits of turning a conference presentation into a published work, it is not yet routine practice. The sheer volume of conference presentations in relation to the number of publications suggests that, for reasons many and varied, a less than proportionate number of people publish work they have presented at conferences. One example of this is the Third International Nurse Education Conference held in Sydney in 2010. Although 216 papers were presented, only 75 (less than 30%) were submitted for publication to the Special Conference Issue of *Nurse Education Today/Nurse Education in Practice (NETNEP) 2010*.

Ethical considerations

It is important to consider publication ethics and copyright provisions relevant to conference proceedings. A conference proceeding refers to a written account of the conference and generally includes all or most of the papers presented. Not all conferences have a book of proceedings and when they do they vary in style. A paper written for a conferencing proceeding book may be a report of the whole presentation or just a synopsis of the key results. Irrespectively, it is meant to be a coherent standalone piece of work that readers can make sense of even if they did not attend the presentation.

Copyright refers to the right to exclusive publication, production and distribution of work such as written papers and conference proceedings. If a conference paper is not published in the proceedings the author retains the copyright and can submit the content without any changes to a journal. In some situations, however, the copyright is transferred to the conference sponsor organisation, which then has the exclusive right to publish that piece of work. If you have transferred the copyright to the conference sponsor organisation, written permission is required before the article can be published in its current form. The copyright owner will usually grant permission for you to publish the work in a peer-reviewed journal. While this approach is not common with nursing conferences, it is important to clarify these types of issues when deciding to present at a conference or publish from that work (see Chapter 12 for issues of publishing ethics).

The barriers to turning the conference paper into publishable work

Writing is easy. All you do is stare at a blank sheet of paper until drops of blood form on your forehead.

Gene Fowler

Finding the time to write is frequently the most challenging part of the publication process, especially if you work in busy clinical environments or demanding academic positions. There is no magic solution other than to allocate your time according to your priorities and values. If publishing is really important to you but you are not giving it priority then you may need to reconsider your time management and learn to curb a tendency to procrastinate. Ask yourself, on a scale of 1–10, how good would you feel if you managed to publish a paper, then ask yourself, on the same scale, how committed you are to achieving this. Do these numbers match?

All of us procrastinate at some time or another, but between 15 and 20% of adults routinely put off activities that would best be done as soon as possible (Gura, 2009). Lack of confidence, overestimating the difficulty of the task and viewing the activity as boring or unpleasant are major reasons for delaying writing. Frequently, people who doubt their ability to write have a worse opinion of their work than anyone else does. For some, negative criticism received in the past might lead to inertia and failure to progress.

Other barriers to turning conference papers into publications may be the initial absence of a plan to do so, not having ethics clearance for the research and leaving the process too long following the presentation. Clinical nurses may not be familiar with the process of submitting a paper and may lack the necessary support. However, there are ways to address many of these issues. Writing support groups may exist in your area, or you could ask your colleagues if they know an academic or experienced writer/researcher interested in your field, with whom you could work.

Strategies for success

A writing project that seems huge and overwhelming is hard to start; breaking it into manageable chunks makes it more achievable. With a distant deadline you are more likely to delay, so set a target date and build in rewards for yourself for meeting timelines. If inclined to procrastinate you should make these deadlines very specific (Gura, 2009): for example 'I will send my draft to my co-author by 6 pm on Friday'. When you meet these deadlines, celebrate, give yourself a pat on the back and plan your next step.

Activity 1   Dealing with procrastination

Record all the reasons why you are delaying turning your conference paper into a published work; be honest, and highlight those related to procrastination.

I have delayed writing this paper because:
  (1)
  (2)
  (3)

If you can argue decisively against your reasons you will be able to start the task. Now write down as convincingly as possible all your arguments against delaying.

I should no longer delay because:

   (1)
   (2)
   (3)

If lack of confidence is your problem, practise positive self-talk with statements such as *I did talk at the conference; I can publish a paper; it does not have to be perfect first time*. Assure yourself that speaking at a conference to peers and strangers takes courage and determination, and that these attributes will see you through the writing and publication process. Further, remind yourself that if your paper was a success at a conference then it is likely to succeed with a wider audience.

Developing effective collaboration with others, especially those with more experience, is an excellent way to start to write. Oermann (2003) suggests that co-authors should appoint a coordinator to monitor progress and keep the group on track. Decisions about authorship and contributions should be made at the beginning of the writing stage; delaying until just before submission can cause tension and hard feelings.

It is not easy to distance yourself from your work: seeking feedback is vital. Be as specific as possible – do you want advice on the style, the structure or the technical content? The one you ask to look at the technical side of the paper is perhaps not the most qualified to advise you about style and grammar: choose the best person to help with each step.

Chief among reasons for procrastination is the misconception that you have to write a perfect piece of work the first time. The advice of Bernard (in Cleary and Walter, 2004) to 'write quickly and edit slowly' is helpful in getting started. It is also a mistake to think that writing is a simple, linear process that follows clearly ordered steps. In reality, as drafts evolve, more thinking and research may lead you to revise your ideas and even the central concepts of the paper or presentation.

Start with the end in mind

Perhaps the most useful advice we can offer is to start with the end in mind: structure, and develop your conference paper and publication concurrently. Once your conference abstract is accepted, decide on an appropriate journal for a linked publication on that topic. Just as you have to meet guidelines for abstracts at conference presentations, you must also be familiar with and adhere to journal's aims and guidelines. Consider well-known journals with a high impact factor: even if your paper is not accepted in the first instance the feedback will be valuable. If you then decide to re-submit to another journal, be sure to observe the style guidelines: Cleary and Walter (2004) point out that editors are quick to detect papers that conform to the style of another journal (see Chapters 2, 5 and 10 for issues related to this and all other aspects of writing for publication).

The following section exemplifies the manner in which a conference paper was turned into a published work by 'starting with the end in mind'.

Conference: 'Getting it right – acute care'. Australian College of Hunter Mental Health Nurses Conference

Conference themes: Acute care, the nature of mental health nursing

Title slide (Figure 9.1):

Warning: This job contains coarse language, violence, nudity, drug use, sexually explicit material and adult themes (and scenes which may offend some nurses)

Teresa Stone and Scott Davis

Figure 9.1 A challenging conference presentation title.

Converting this conference paper into a published work needed careful consideration and a number of changes. While the paper relied for its impact on verbal and visual techniques, the punchy title, suitable for a conference, would not translate to an effective journal title wherein key words play a greater role. Adapting the abstract (Box 9.1) for publication meant making the subject of the paper explicit, honing in to the key messages and writing the abstract according to the dictates of the Journal – in this case the *International Journal of Mental Health Nursing*.

Both the presentation and the published paper were discussion papers. Adaptation to a published work required omission of the more speculative material; the tone of the published paper was more serious than the conference presentation, in which humour was used to convey what was essentially a very serious message and the audiences differed. The conference audience were familiar with the presenters and the context of practice and were relatively homogeneous. Readership of the journal is international, so the context (Australia) had to be made more explicit.

Scientific committees for conferences and journal editors use different review criteria. Acceptance for a conference depends upon the quality of the abstract, alignment with conference themes, breadth of coverage of particular topics and the balance between clinical and research papers. The review process tends to be less rigorous, as the decision is based on the

Box 9.1

Conference abstract: Acute mental health nursing necessarily means exposure to offensive and, sometimes, highly offensive material and events, and mental health nurses work with people who have experienced many extreme emotional traumas. Exposure to verbal aggression alone has been linked with feelings of distress, anger, powerlessness, job dissatisfaction, depersonalisation and emotional exhaustion in nurses, and vicarious trauma is increasingly recognised as an issue for clinicians. One challenge of nursing in an acute setting is to maintain one's sense of self without withdrawing from patient contact or losing therapeutic optimism. This creates an intrinsic paradox between the general view of nursing as a caring profession and the reality of nursing in acute mental health settings in a contemporary society. This complex and challenging environment requires nurses who work in these settings to develop robust personal and organisational strategies to deal with this reality.

This paper will discuss the contention that, in order to get it right, mental health nurses cannot deny the reality of what 'it' – the acute mental health environment – presents. To this end, mental health nurses must be prepared professionally, mentally, ethically and morally to deal with coarse language, violence, nudity, drug use, sexually explicit material and adult themes.

quality of the abstract alone. By contrast, journal papers are accepted following blind review of the full paper by two or more reviewers. This means that you will have to present a coherent, well-structured paper, which is grounded in relevant literature.

The conference paper outlined previously was transformed into a published work and the manuscript submitted and accepted for publication. Developing the conference paper and the manuscript was a concurrent process. The title of the publication is: An overview of swearing and its impact on mental health nursing practice (Stone and Hazelton, 2008) (Box 9.2).

Activity 2   Planning a conference paper and journal publication concurrently

Select a conference for which you plan to submit an abstract and identify the conference themes.
Identify an appropriate journal, whose aims and scope accord with conference themes, to which you would like to submit the paper.
List the journal aims and read the journal guidelines.
Prepare an abstract for the conference.
Re-write the abstract to conform with the journal guidelines and aims.

Box 9.2

Journal abstract: Swearing is a subject largely ignored in academic circles but impossible to ignore in the workplace. Nurses encounter swearing from patients and their carers, staff and managers and use swear words in communication with each other. Language is the major tool of the mental health nurse, and swearing is an aspect of language frequently used in situations of intense emotion. This paper provides an overview of the historical, legal and cultural aspects of swearing in an Australian context in order to assist nurses in their practice.

Key words: communication, dialectical behaviour therapy, language, swearing, therapeutic relationship, verbal behaviour.

The title

The title is one of the most important aspects of writing and presenting but can be decided upon once you have completed your abstract. The title influences whether your presentation will be attended and your publication read. Choose it with your audience in mind and make it powerful enough to attract readers, yet simple and clear enough to appeal to them. The functions of a title are to capture the reader's interest, clarify the specific content of the work and reflect its approach. For conferences your title should both excite and inform potential readers. Attention grabbers include:

- *A question*: 'Is simulation an effective replacement for clinical placements'?
- *Alliteration*: 'Fast food fuss: Nurses and nutrition'.
- *Wordplay*: 'Back to swear one: understanding swearwords'.
- *A phrase currently in the news, applying it to your work*: 'Shock and awe: The impact of swearing on nurses'.

Titles for publications, while capturing the reader's attention, should also conform to publishing conventions. The title for a journal should indicate the subject or clinical problem and method of enquiry; and for research papers the design should be included, for example 'Coping with chronic pain: A questionnaire survey'. Review papers should also be evident from the title, for example 'Patient empowerment: A literature review'.

Activity 3   Selecting a title

Review conference proceedings and journal articles and take note of the titles and abstracts that attract your attention.

List three ideas specific to your topic that would capture your audience's/readers' attention.

Write a title for your conference presentation and one for your publication.

The introduction

Just like a journal article, a conference paper requires an introduction, body and conclusion. You will capture your listeners' attention by beginning with a question, a funny story, a profound statistic, a startling comment or something that will make them think. It is then usual to state your purpose or present an outline of your talk. The slide that follows your title slide usually outlines the key points to be covered. For example, see Figure 9.2.

Overview

- The classifiable elements of our work
- Prevalence of swearing
- Preliminary results
- Therapeutics implications of swearing
- Implications for policy and practice

Figure 9.2   Stating the content of the conference presentation.

This presentation overview became the draft of an introduction to the journal paper (Box 9.3).

Activity 4   Planning your presentation and introduction

Design the second slide of your presentation.

Begin with a bullet point plan of the aims and key points of your presentation.

Next, draft an introduction for your journal manuscript based upon these key points.

Developing your presentation and manuscript concurrently

Effective presentation requires the content and structure to be adjusted to the medium of speech; we can use images, voice tone, body language and eye

Box 9.3

Introduction: Nurses are regularly exposed to swearing by patients and carers and from professional colleagues. Given the extent of such exposure, it is surprising that no literature exists on this aspect of nursing practice in general and mental health nursing in particular. In this paper, we will take swearing to mean language use in which the expression: (1) refers to something that is taboo and/or stigmatised in the culture; (2) [may] not be interpreted literally and (3) can be used to express strong emotions and attitudes (Andersson and Trudgill, 1990, p. 53). Defining features of swearing are its capacity to shock because of its association with a tabooed object and the vital role it plays in both normal and abnormal communication (Van Lancker, 1990). In what follows, we begin by briefly discussing the historical and legal aspects of swearing before examining gender and legal issues; the paper will then shift to a discussion of how swearing is responded to in the clinical setting, with implications for nursing practice. While much of what is argued may apply to other countries, the paper focuses especially on the Australian context (Stone and Hazelton, 2008).

contact to convey our message. Asking questions of your audience secures their attention so that they are engaged and actively listening. You can also illustrate your presentation with stories and personal experiences. These techniques, so effective for an oral presentation, may not translate directly into a publishable paper, and for this reason a different and more formal stylistic approach is needed.

To save yourself the laborious task of going over the same ground twice, we suggest that when preparing your conference presentation you write complete notes, fully referenced, for each PowerPoint slide. They will be useful in preparing for the presentation but will also facilitate later writing of you manuscript for publication. Begin with bullet points; then add some detail. When preparing your paper you can use these bullet points to structure your paper. For example, see Figure 9.3 and Box 9.4.

Activity 5   Developing and finalising your manuscript for submission

Using the above example, develop your presentation with full notes for each slide.

Expand on these bullet points to develop your manuscript.

Seek peer review of your draft manuscript.

Refer to the checklist at the end of this chapter for guidance.

Limitations

- It is highly probable that, as in other studies, aggression and verbal aggression were under-reported.

- Nurses who were likely to be more offended may have declined to participate or withdrawn from the study.

Figure 9.3 Key issues to note in discussion.

Box 9.4

Notes page for slide 28 - Limitations

(1) Personal, interpersonal, cultural and sub-cultural factors tend to and will continue to influence the degree to which incidents are recorded.

(2) Highly probable that aggression and especially verbal aggression were underreported. Anecdotally this is the case; for example the psychiatric emergency centre has only one documented incident of aggression for a year. *Ask the audience if they record verbal aggression in their facilities.* Perhaps it is reported only when accompanied by physical aggression. Underreporting also may occur because aggressive behaviour tends to occur in clusters; nurses may not have the time to complete the Modified Overt Aggression Scale (MOAS) after every incident (Sorgi et al., 1991). Nurses may believe that there is no point in recording verbal aggression (VA) because reporting does not lead to positive changes.

(3) Anecdotally, staff working on particular units in the present study report that levels of verbal aggression and swearing are so high that not only are they not reported but staff have also ceased to register the behaviour as verbal aggression. It is unclear why a reduction in the severity of verbal aggression may have occurred in 2004.

(4) It has been calculated that up to five times as many assaults were perpetrated against psychiatric inpatient staff than were formally reported (Arboleda-Florez et al., 1994).

Writing the conclusion

In the same way that the overview slide of your presentation can be used to develop the abstract of your publication, the 'take home message' of your presentation can be used to develop the conclusion of your paper. You need to conclude your presentation by summarising the main points to ensure that the audience understands and remembers your key messages. When crafting the conclusion of your paper the same approach is needed. For example, see Figure 9.4.

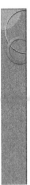

In summary

- Dealing with the extremes of human emotion and behaviour is central to the work of acute means health nurses.
- Clinicians need to have a better understanding of the socio-cultural aspects of swearing.
- Support and debriefing should be readily available for distressing levels of verbal aggression.
- Health policies on aggression need to be mindful of the clinical needs of patients as well as the safety of staff.

Figure 9.4 Key messages for conference audience and final paper.

Timeline

From the drafting and submission of a conference abstract to the publication of an article can be a 12–18-month process that requires careful

> **Box 9.5 Conclusion in the published paper**
>
> A better understanding of the role played by swearing, culturally, developmentally and in relation to mental health disorders, is likely to lead to improvements in the therapeutic relationship between nurses and their patients and thus have positive effects on treatment outcomes. This paper has outlined ways in which the emotional content of swearing can be dealt with more strategically. The experience of being sworn at and exposed to swearing is common to all mental health nurses. It is time to move beyond treating swearing in punitive ways and to look for the therapeutic opportunities that are inherent in all verbal exchanges between nurses and patients (Stone and Hazelton, 2008).

Table 9.2 Important milestones to achieve successful presentation, writing and publication.

Task	Date
Conference announcement.	
Call for abstracts.	
Ascertain means of support for conference attendance (financial and study leave).	
Select topic – How will your paper fit in with the main topics and themes?	
Identify co-presenters/co-authors (if you are a research candidate you will need to discuss this with your supervisors).	
Write (and re-write) the abstract, seeking consensus with co-presenters/co-authors.	
Submit abstract (usually an online process).	
Date of notification of abstract acceptance (or otherwise).	
Apply for support for conference attendance (financial and study leave).	
Begin to draft presentation (using bullet points) working collaboratively with your co-authors and/or supervisors.	
For each slide write notes (this will later be used for your paper).	
Finalise the conference paper and the notes pages. Ensure consensus with co-authors/supervisors on the final paper.	
Send PowerPoint presentation to the conference organisers.	
Present the paper and celebrate!	
Reflect on and record any feedback received from the audience.	
Discuss the feedback with co-authors/supervisors and make changes to the notes pages.	
Begin to re-draft the paper in according to the journal aims and guidelines seeking consensus and working collaboratively with co-authors.	
Finalise paper and seek agreement of co-authors.	
Submit paper and wait for decision.	
Celebrate your achievement!	

planning. The material you present at a conference is frequently a 'work in progress' and may be nowhere near as polished as a journal article requires, so allow yourself time to ensure that your work is of a standard that journal requires.

> ### Activity 6
>
> Complete Table 9.2, identifying the important milestones in developing your timeline for writing, presenting at an upcoming conference and publishing your paper.

Conclusion

...Writing is hard work (whether a conference paper or a published work). One has to sit down on that chair and think and transform thoughts into readable, consecutive, interesting sentences that both make sense and make the reader turn the page. It is laborious, slow, often painful, sometimes agony. It means rearrangement, revision, adding, cutting, rewriting. But it brings about a sense of excitement, almost of rapture; a moment on Olympus. In short, it is an act of creation.

Barbara Tuchman

We hope that we have persuaded you of the value of getting 'two in one' and walked you through the process of turning a conference paper into publishable work. While conference papers can circulate widely through informal networks, usually the impact on the advancement of knowledge is small and if you want to have a larger impact, it is important to follow up with a journal article. Presenting gives you the opportunity to 'test drive' your work with audiences that represent a microcosm of the audience who will be reading your article. The goal of turning your conference paper into a published work gives you incentive, a deadline and is a valuable first step to becoming a published author. When you have achieved this success, reflect on the process, what you have learnt, your next goal and how you can use your insights to support other potential writers.

References

Andersson, L. & Trudgill, P. (1990) *Bad Language*. Oxford: Blackwell Publishing Ltd.

Arboleda-Florez, J., Crisanti, A., Rose, S. & Holley, H. (1994) Measuring aggression on psychiatric inpatient units: development and testing of the Calgary General Hospital Aggression Scale. *International Journal of Offender Therapy and Comparative Criminology*, 38, 183–204.

Baldwin, C. & Chandler, G.E. (2002) Improving faculty publication output: the role of a writing coach. *Journal of Professional Nursing*, 18(1), 8–15.

Cleary, M. & Walter, G. (2004) Apportioning our time and energy: oral presentation, poster, journal article or other? *International Journal of Mental Health Nursing*, 13, 204–207.

Dixon, N. (2001) Writing for publication – a guide for new authors. *International Journal for Quality in Health Care*, 13(5), 417–421.

Gura, T. (2009) I'll do it tomorrow. *Scientific American*, December 2008/January 2009, 27–33.

Lee, A. & Boud, D. (2003) Writing groups, change and academic identity: research development as local practice. *Studies in Higher Education*, 28(2), 187–200.

Murray, R. & Newton, M. (2008) Facilitating writing for publication. *Physiotherapy*, 94(1), 29–34.

Oermann, M.H. (2003) Sharing your work: building knowledge about nursing care quality. *Journal of Nursing Care Quality*, 18, 243–244.

Savitz, D.A. (2000) Failure to publish results of epidemiologic studies is unethical. *Epidemiology*, 11(3), 361–363.

Sorgi, P., Ratey, J., Knoedler, D.W., Markert, R.J. & Reichman, M. (1991) Rating aggression in the clinical setting, a retrospective adaptation of the Overt Aggression Scale: preliminary results. *Journal of Neuropsychiatry*, 3, 552–556.

Stone, T.E. & Hazelton, M. (2008) An overview of swearing and its impact on mental health nursing practice. *International Journal of Mental Health Nursing*, 17, 208–214.

Stone, T., Levett-Jones, T., Harris, M. & Sinclair, P. (2010) The genesis of the neophyte writers' group. *Nurse Education Today*, 30, 657–661.

Taylor, J., Lyon, P. & Harris, J. (2005) Writing for publication: a new skill for nurses? *Nurse Education in Practice*, 5(2), 91–96.

VanEvery, J. (2011) Do conference papers count? *Jo VanEvery: Helping you be a better academic*. Available at: http://jovanevery.ca/conference-papers-value/ [Accessed 23 April 2012].

Van Lancker, D. (1990) The neurology of proverbs. *Behavioural Neurology*, 3, 169–187.

Winslow, E.H. (1996) Failure to publish research: a form of scientific misconduct? *Heart & Lung: Journal of Acute & Critical Care*, 25(3), 169–171.

Winslow, S.A., Mullaly, L.M. & Blankenship, J.S. (2008) You should publish that: helping staff nurses get published. *Nursing for Women's Health*, 12, 120–126.

Further reading

Hartley, J. (2008) *Academic Writing and Publishing – A Practical Handbook*, Abingdon: Routledge.

Saver, C. (2011) *Anatomy of Writing for Publication for Nurses*, Indianapolis, IN, Sigma Theta Tau International.

Websites

A number of links to papers on conference abstracts and reporting. Available at: http://www.oup.com/uk/orc/bin/9780199563104/01student/chapters/ch10/references/[Accessed 8 June 2012].

Chapter 10

The Editorial Process

Roger Watson

Faculty of Health and Social Care, University of Hull, Hull, UK

Introduction

Given that you may be considering writing an article for publication it is helpful to understand the editorial process, that is the role that editors have and the journey of your manuscript from submission to publication. This will also help you to understand the submission process and how you and the editorial team manage your manuscript once you have submitted it. The more you know about this, the more knowledgeable you can be in any interaction with the editor or other staff on the journal. If you have aspirations to become an editor then this chapter may help you to decide and inform any future decisions. You may also have been invited to become an associate editor of a journal or a guest editor for a special issue of the journal focusing on your area of expertise.

Who are editors?

The editors of this book are both editors for journals published by leading international publishers, and the chapter authors include several other editors. Editors are often seen as people who are remote from the daily work of researching and writing manuscripts for publication but nothing could be further from the truth and some editors are very keen to share their experiences, as one, describing herself in a blog as FemaleScienceProfessor, has done (http://science-professor.blogspot.com/; Accessed 7 December 2011). Others such as Miser (1998) have shared their perspective on the role and Hames (2007) has written an excellent book outlining the peer-review and manuscript management process based on many years of experience. These are all excellent resources to help you understand the process of editing.

Most editors are hired after an application and interview process or actually invited by publishing companies, both to lead and partly to manage a

Writing for Publication in Nursing and Healthcare: Getting It Right, First Edition.
Edited by Karen Holland and Roger Watson.
© 2012 John Wiley & Sons, Ltd. Published 2012 by John Wiley & Sons, Ltd.

Box 10.1 Finding out more about editors

Check the journal websites of a few major nursing journals and open up any links that refer you to the 'Editorial Board'. Take a look at the people involved and ask yourself the following questions:

- What kind of people assume the role of Editor-in-Chief (if a journal has one)?
- Who are the editors; why do you think they have been invited to assume this role?
- Do all editors do the same job?
- Does every journal follow the same pattern for the jobs undertaken by editors?
- What purpose do you think the editorial board serves?

particular journal. Generally, they are experienced and well-published academics in their own right with considerable experience in academic publishing gained over many years serving on editorial boards and in other editorial positions. Therefore, they are like you in many ways, they understand what it is like to be writing and submitting manuscripts to journals and they also know how much effort it takes to get published and the sense of achievement it brings.

However, they also know the standards that are required in terms of scholarship in their subject as well as being committed to disseminating high-quality publications and the development of authorship skill and standards. They often seek to work in academic publishing because they wish to see these skills and standards preserved. Try the activity in Box 10.1, which is designed to help you find out more about the kind of people who are editors and the range of jobs they undertake with the journals.

What is editing about?

Some of the technical aspects of editing will be reviewed here but the role is not simply about receiving manuscripts, making decisions and editing your writing. A great deal of the role of an editor is, in association with the publisher, managing the day-to-day running of the journal, ensuring that 'the copy' (that is, manuscripts submitted, those in the system and those that get finally get published) flows smoothly and that accepted manuscripts are published within a reasonable time following acceptance. In addition, editors deal with authors' and readers' enquiries, and with infringements of publication ethics such as possible plagiarism or copyright issues (see Chapter 12).

It is always worth considering contacting an editor if you are thinking about submitting a manuscript to a journal and you are not sure if it will really meet the standards or the aims and scope of the journal. Sometimes the editor's email will be provided on the journal web page or you will be directed to the email address of the editorial office from where your enquiry will be directed to an editor.

Frequently, editors will be well known and may be contacted via their work email, but it is more advisable to use the route advertised on the journal web page as the enquiry will be logged and your details recorded in case you do not hear from someone in a reasonable time. Editors are not normally working full time as an editor of a journal, most work part-time or full time in other roles and manage the editor role in addition to this work.

If you do make an enquiry about a manuscript to a journal, it is always advisable to send an abstract, presented in the style of the journal, or as some authors do, send a draft outline. It is usually not advisable to send a complete manuscript as editors will rarely have time to read a full manuscript at the enquiry stage and will easily be able to make a decision based on a well-written abstract if the proposed article meets firstly, the aims and scope of the journal and secondly, whether it has potential as a publication.

Who else is involved?

Editors do not normally work alone; as noted previously they are hired normally on fixed-term contracts by publishing companies who will also publish a range of journals and who will offer varying levels of support to their journal offices and editors. The two key roles that are important for you to understand as a potential author are (1) the Editor-in-Chief and (2) the editor roles. Other members of the publishing team will be considered later in the chapter.

The Editor-in-Chief

On the major well-established academic journals there will usually be a team of editors led by an Editor-in-Chief, for example *The Journal of Advanced Nursing*. The Editor-in-Chief role varies between journals. Most Editors-in-Chief will have had considerable experience in academic publishing and a long association with publishing companies. In some cases, they play a purely leadership role: helping to set journal policy, promoting the journal internationally and liaising with the publisher. Others will be more engaged in the daily running of the journal and, in addition to the above roles, will also be engaged in editing the manuscripts that are published. At some point in the process, it is usual for the Editor-in-Chief to select the manuscripts that are assigned to editors, to edit the final copy of manuscripts or to compile issues of the journal, that is select the articles that will be published in each issue. In some cases, the Editor-in-Chief will play a major 'gate-keeping' role by deciding which manuscripts will proceed to review. Manuscripts that do not fit the aims and scope of the journal (see Chapter 5), which appear to add little to the field of knowledge and those that do not fit the submission criteria – if not already 'filtered out' by the editorial assistant (see Section 'What happens to your manuscript?') – will simply be rejected at this stage. Those that are deemed suitable for review will either be allocated directly to reviewers or allocated to an editor for further consideration, and either rejection by them or allocation to reviewers. In other international journals, this role of Editor-in-Chief is undertaken by the editor, who undertakes the same responsibilities outlined here for their journal. They may, however, have associate editors with specific responsibilities for other editorial roles on the journal team, such as Book Review Editor (see Chapter 4).

Tip 1

It is worth reiterating here the importance of reading and following the guidelines for the journal. A major cause of rejection in the early stages of submission is that manuscripts have not followed some crucial aspect of the guidance, either on the process of submission or in the presentation of the manuscript. See Chapters 2 and 5 to remind yourself of how important it is to follow journal guidelines. See Box 10.2 for an exercise related to the guidance on submission.

Editors

In a journal where there is an Editor-in-Chief, the real work of editing or managing the daily routine of article submission and process lies with those editors who will assign reviewers to their manuscripts and then receive the reviews and arrive at a decision in terms of revision, rejection or acceptance. Before

---

Box 10.2 The submission process

Check the web pages of a few journals, especially from different publishers, and compare and contrast the guidance on the submission process. See if you can find answers to the following questions:
- Do all journals use the same online submission process?
- Should you have enquired to the journal about the suitability of your manuscript prior to submission?
- Are tables and figures always submitted separately from the main text?
- Is it necessary to assign copyright on submission?
- Do all authors need to sign the copyright form?
- Does the journal require a covering letter?
- To what other points about the submission process should you pay attention?

they finally decide to accept a manuscript they will have to read it carefully and edit it to make it clearer and more concise, to comply with house style and to make sure that the writing is acceptable. However, in terms of house style, some journals use copy editors to deal with the technical aspects of writing and the editor's role is simply to make decisions on suitability for publication. Again this is very much dependent on the publishers expectations and the guidance they may give the authors in terms of any further amendments.

Often, they will request that the author makes some final changes, some of which will have been suggested by reviewers, and they will issue a final check-list for the author to refer to prior to the final submission of the accepted manuscript. This is rarely the end of the editing process; in some cases, the editor will take a final look at the manuscript prior to sending it to the pro-duction section of the publishing company; sometimes this final edit will be undertaken by the Editor-in-Chief.

Therefore, the manuscript that is sent to production and eventually pub-lished will usually differ from the one originally submitted. It is very important that you should understand this and take the view that each step in this pro-cess is being carried out by people with considerable experience and that each step in the process is an improvement; the final manuscript is a team effort. The key member in the team of course still being you as the author of the paper and there will still be a further role for you to play later in the editorial process, that is the checking of the final proofs of the article prior to publication, either electronically or in paper format.

A typical chart for the flow of copy is shown in Figure 10.1.

What do editors look for in an article?

Editors ensure that each paper accepted for publication in their journal is of the highest quality possible and one way of ensuring this is to eliminate or reject papers that are of manifestly poor quality, irrelevant to the aims and scope of the journal and unlikely to survive the review process. This is one of the major challenges for the editor, as this means that every article that is submitted has to be read by one of the journal editors or Editor-in-Chief to maintain the high standards expected of the journal.

Editors will also be looking out for papers that are likely to be read and cited and, thereby, improve or maintain the journal's standing in the publishing community. This takes place on submission to the journal, and it will depend on how much space the editor has to fill and how much material is being submitted as to how decisions are made at this stage.

It is logical that when there is plenty of copy (the general publishing indus-try term for what is submitted, processed and published) – which is usually synonymous with being a high-quality journal, that editors will be more se-lective, and vice versa. Likewise, depending on the volume of submissions, decisions on receiving reviews from the reviewers (see Chapter 11) will be ad-justed to take into account the need to fill the available space. Therefore, in a

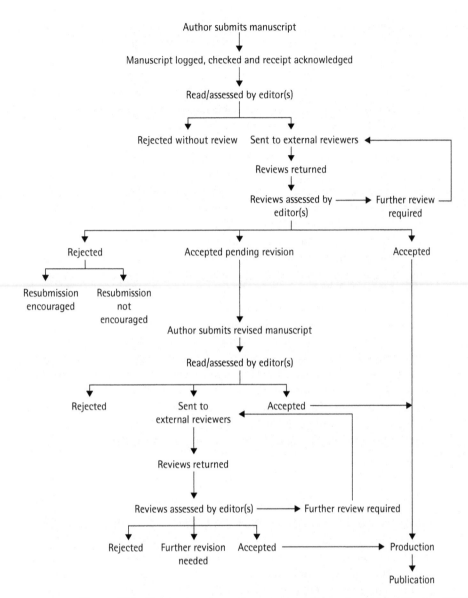

Figure 10.1 The basic peer-review process. (Reproduced from Hames, 2007.)

high-quality journal receiving a high volume of manuscripts, decisions are likely to be harsher at this stage and the rejection rate will be higher. Therefore, what editors are looking for is the best possible quality article from the onset of the submission, and taking other considerations such as possible themed issues, into account. One of the reasons that this book came about, was our recognition of the need to support potential new authors as well as those who may be experiencing a high rejection rate from journals.

Beyond regulating the flow of 'copy', editors are then concerned with taking each manuscript that is submitted for publication and making sure that it meets the standards of the journal. This is more than simply meeting the house style and conventions, although experienced editors usually have a keen eye for that. Editors also like to ensure that the writing is as clear and concise as possible; essentially, the manuscripts will conform to a certain 'style' that is characteristic of the editor and the journal. The term 'Plain English' is often used for this clarity and conciseness of language and structure.

Style is very hard to define but the general style of academic papers is to eliminate individual style as far as possible, and the idiosyncrasies, empty phrases and additional words that many people use unconsciously will usually be removed at this stage. This is not the same as removing the content of the article or interference with the actual meaning of findings or discussion, for example. This is about ensuring good practice in structure and language that will be understood by the international reader. If, however, there is lack of clarity around content of the article, which affects the general style or structure, then the reviewers normally pick that up in the review process as does the editor, who will then communicate that concern and query to the authors.

This editing to an accepted style is not meant to demonstrate the superiority of the editor or the stupidity of the author; editors are authors too and their published work will go through the same process. The point is to sharpen the focus of the manuscript and avoid ambiguity. The fewer points that editors have to change in your work the more impressed they will be with you writing. We have adopted this same principle in the writing of this book, because the same strictures lead us to ensure some degree of conformity with language and style, but allowing for individual thought and approach to the overall way the chapters are written. This is comparable to editing an article.

Editorial boards

Academic journals always have editorial boards and, like editors, their role varies across journals and publishers. Editorial boards are appointed by the publisher – usually on the advice of the editors, to advise the editor and publishers about developments and trends in the field of interest of the journal. Methods of appointment and terms of office of editorial board members vary. In some journals the editor or Editor-in-Chief will chair the editorial board and, essentially, lead them in their role; for other journals the editorial board is chaired by the publisher or a member of the board appointed as chair and the Editor-in-Chief is accountable to the board for the management of the journal and the publications. In some cases, the editorial board is relatively small and the journal will appoint a series of advisers to the board, for example in *Ageing and Society* (http://agingandsociety.com/ideas/advisory-board/; Accessed 23 April 2012); in other cases, the board itself is larger. For some journals the editorial board and the reviewers for the journal are the same people but for others, the editorial board members may be reviewers but the journal will draw on a much wider pool of expertise, who make up the Panel of Reviewers.

Box 10.3   Editorial boards

Check the URLs provided in the paragraphs in the previous text and compare and contrast the composition and work of different editorial boards.

The highly cited and prestigious journal *Nature* has no editorial board; instead, a team of professional editors make all decisions regarding the journal (http://www.nature.com/nature/about/editors/; Accessed 23 April 2012).

Commonly, editorial board members come from many countries and they can provide advice specific to their region as well as either an academic or a clinical speciality area. The specific responsibilities of editorial board members vary but they may be expected to review manuscripts, write editorials and provide feedback on any proposals for developing the journal. There are no specific qualifications for editorial board membership, but being well published and eminent in your field is one route. However, clinical expertise and specific knowledge (e.g. statistics) is also important. Many journals, such as *Nurse Education in Practice* will have a small international editorial board but also have a much larger international advisory board who give advice on regional issues, support the journal at conferences and most importantly, are also members of the Panel of Reviewers.

Whatever editorial board system is in place, the key factor for any journal that states that it is an international journal is that this is visible in the way it conducts its editorial board role and supports international dialogue and networking. To enable you to consider this role further and how it has an impact on the aims and scope of the journal and therefore your article submission, try the activity in Box 10.3, of accessing and reviewing the way journal editorial boards are set up and what their role is.

What happens to your manuscript?

When you submit a manuscript to a journal (most major publishers now have an electronic submission process but others will still be requesting other forms of submission), there will be a filtering process to ensure that your manuscript is suitable for the journal.

An initial inspection of the manuscript will be carried out by an editorial assistant or administration editor, often a full time employee of the publishing company, to ensure that there are no viruses in the files that you submitted and that, on a cursory inspection, the manuscript is written in reasonably good English, that the manuscript is within the word length permitted by the journal and that it conforms to other conventions of the journal. In addition, they take note of any specific information that the author wishes the editor to know about in their submission letter.

If the manuscript meets the above specifications then it will be passed on to an editor or the Editor-in-Chief for a decision about its suitability for further processing by editors and reviewers (Hames, 2007). At this stage, an editor or the Editor-in-Chief will consider the potential of the manuscript to survive the review process but also how well it suits the journal, the likelihood of it being read and cited and whether it is sufficiently novel to merit publication. At this point, it should be noted that editors and Editors-in-Chief are taking a risk and exercising their judgement; they do not always 'get it right', as some manuscripts that are rejected at this stage – and, indeed, further on in the process – are published by other journals and then highly cited there. Of course, it is important to note that these articles will have had to be revised prior to submission to other journals.

If the manuscript is rejected at this stage then the Editor-in-Chief/editor will merely indicate that the manuscript is not a priority for the journal, it does not meet the aims and scope or that it has not been submitted to the right journal. They may sometimes recommend another journal and thank you for submitting it and for showing an interest in the journal. Usually, further feedback on the manuscript will not be provided.

At this stage there is usually no right of appeal against the Editor-in-Chief's decision but there is nothing to stop you contacting the journal if you think you have been badly treated or you believe that an obvious mistake has been made. It is very rare that experienced editors will change their mind at this stage but ensure that the author is contacted with the same advice as previously. For manuscripts that the Editor-in-Chief consider worthy of passing on to an editor or the reviewers, the editor will also scrutinise it and may also take a decision to reject at this stage.

Usually on those journals where there are these two levels of editorial decision-making (e.g. see *Journal of Clinical Nursing*) the editors will have responsibility for a section of the journal or for a particular type of manuscript and will look at the manuscripts from that perspective. If the editor is satisfied that the manuscript is suitable then it will be sent to reviewers for expert opinion on the manuscript. Reviewing is covered in Chapter 11 but, from the editorial perspective, it is well recognised that reviewing is a capricious process; that is, pairs of reviewers (in the normal double- blind peer-review process) can normally agree on a decision, albeit with slight variation in what they consider is required of the article, but it is also possible for reviewers to be diametrically opposed in their opinion on a manuscript. For example one reviewer can recommend accepting a manuscript without changes while another can recommend rejection (Hames, 2007).

The editor then has to make a decision to convey to the author; the decision conveyed to the author may reflect both or neither of the individual decisions of the reviewers but a judgement that takes both views into account and allows the author to revise the manuscript accordingly, or they may on reading it themselves issue a rejection. Usually, the editor will simply convey a decision along with the comments and leave the author to decide how best to address these but, sometimes, the editor will advise on the best path to take. The best advice for authors is, if in any doubt about the reviewer and editorial feedback sent to them, is to consult with the editor about the best course of action.

Where is my manuscript?

Once you have submitted your manuscript you may be anxious to know what stage in the editorial and reviewing process the manuscript has reached. This is definitely an enquiry for the editorial office and not the Editor-in-Chief. Journals commonly provide an online tracking facility for manuscripts and this extends beyond the editorial and review process to the production process. You should check this before making any enquiries and then, only if you are clear that the process has been delayed. When you submit an article electronically you are normally given a number and a password where you can track your article in the process. Certainly this has reduced the number of telephone inquiries for many editors, as the authors know exactly where their article is in the system. If, however, they can see that it is taking longer than they consider normal for the journal then they may well contact the editorial office or the editor directly.

Appealing against rejection

It is now considered good practice for journals to have an appeals process against rejection, following the review process, and this appeals process should be specified in the journal web pages or easily obtainable from the editorial offices. To determine exact protocols to be used please see the exercise in Box 10.4.

Dealing with reviewers' comments

As described previously, the decision conveyed to you by the editor will be one that has been taken on the basis of all the comments received from reviewers, and the decision will range from 'reject', in which case you do not need to respond directly to the journal, through major or minor revisions, to accept; the last decision is very rare following a first submission and you may still receive requests to revise following re-submission. Anything is possible, but the more you take account of the advice and guidance we have provided in this book in relation to different forms of publications the better chance there

---

Box 10.4 Journal appeals processes

Check a few journal web pages and see if you can identify an appeals process against rejection. It may be useful to begin with a word/phrase search in Google.

is of being asked to revise the paper for possible publication in your first choice journal. If the article is rejected then you would be wise to take the comments of the reviewers and editor into account in revising the manuscript for submission to another journal – but ensure that you take the time to read the author guidelines of that journal prior to rewriting.

What is important is the way you respond to the comments and the decision you receive, and you may notice that the comments are congruent or they can be disparate. It is unlikely that you will agree with all of the comments of the reviewers but you must give them all serious consideration. Some comments may even be contradictory as there is no collusion between the reviewers who, in addition to being blind to the authors (that is unknown to them) – as you are to them – are also blind to each other.

Where reviewers' comments are contradictory, it is impossible to take a middle road; you will have to decide which comments are the most important with regard to the focus of your paper and the important thing in responding is not to ignore any of the reviewers comments but to address them all, even if your response is to state that you (politely) disagree with the comments or that they cannot be addressed. Almost invariably, this is satisfactory and if you have any fears that you will run into problems having the manuscript accepted, it is appropriate to correspond with the editor directly.

Production of the article

When you have a manuscript accepted by a journal then the manuscript enters the next stage of the editorial process, which is production. Normally, the Editor-in-Chief will have had a final review of the manuscript to ensure that it meets the standards of the journal in terms of content and journal conventions before indicating that the manuscript is ready for production. The production process is not, strictly speaking, under the control of the Editor-in-Chief; however, the Editor-in-Chief will liaise closely with the production team, often led by a production assistant or a production editor and this team is employed directly by the publishing company.

The job of production is to take the raw manuscript, usually in a Word document format, and transform this into the portable document format (pdf) that is a facsimile of the paper that will eventually be published. This is called a proof. In the process of producing the pdf, several checks will be made on the manuscript and the production team will often have '*macros*' – which are ways to automate repeated tasks in word-processing packages – whereby the formatting of the references in the main body of the text and in the list and cross-checking between the two is enabled. Any queries about the pdf will be indicated by number on the proof. Increasingly, comments and alterations can be entered directly on pdfs through the use of computer software programmes, making printing and manual marking up unnecessary.

You may feel that you have been kept waiting a long time during the editorial and reviewing process and that the journal is very demanding towards the end of the process but proofs need to be corrected and returned very quickly after receipt (normally within 48 hours after receipt) and it is important to adhere to any dates given as delays will only hold up the publication of your paper. If you expect that there will be any delays in responding to them then you must keep the production office informed, otherwise you may hold up production of the journal issue or your paper may be substituted by another one and publication of your paper will be severely delayed. However, many journals now have an electronic online version of your article many months prior to it appearing in a paper base version and some issues are completely electronic viewing only (see *Journal of Clinical Nursing* Virtual Issue on Violence: http://onlinelibrary.wiley.com/journal/10.1111/%28ISSN%291365-2702/homepage/virtual_issue_violence.htm; Accessed 4 December 2011).

Digital object identifiers

At the proof stage most journals will assign a number that is unique to the proof and that will follow the proof to publication online and in hard copy and this number is called a digital object identifier (DOI). The number can be found on the first page of the proof and looks like this: (doi: 10.1111/j.1365-2702.2010.03049.x). Here is what the International DOI foundation says about DOIs (http://www.doi.org/; Accessed 15 May 2011):

> The Digital Object Identifier (DOI®) system is for identifying content objects in the digital environment. DOI names are assigned to any entity for use on digital networks. They are used to provide current information, including where they (or information about them) can be found on the Internet. Information about a digital object may change over time, including where to find it, but its DOI name will not change.

The DOI of a paper can be used to locate it online by typing the DOI into a search engine. Most journals publish online early in advance of hard copy issues (see http://www.sciencedirect.com/science/journal/aip/14715953 and http://onlinelibrary.wiley.com/journal/10.1111/(ISSN)1365-2702/earlyview) and a convenient aspect of DOIs is that, once the paper is published online it is fully published and can be cited in other papers and listed in Curriculum Vitae (CVs) as a record of publication.

You should only make corrections to obvious errors at this proof checking stage – and please read it carefully, as they do 'creep in' despite numerous checks by numerous trained people, but this is not the time to make major alterations to your paper; if major alterations are required then the paper should really enter the production stage again. This is costly and, while rare, publishers often reserve the right to charge you at this stage – especially if the major corrections are your fault.

Correcting your own work can be hard and unless mistakes are very obvious, authors can often overlook them. The proof will be read by a member of the production team but if you are in any doubt about your ability to correct your own work – familiarity with the work can be a disadvantage – then ask a colleague, emphasising that this is for correction and not alteration.

Ethics

Editors will be very concerned about publication ethics and will respond to any doubts raised by reviewers or that arise in the process of random checking regarding the authenticity, originality or duplication of the work reported in a manuscript (Hames, 2007). The response will be to investigate any concerns that are raised and act on any adverse findings. Generally speaking, with the advent of electronic publishing and the Internet, it is easier to detect any kind of fraud than it used to be. Specific and very sensitive software is now available and the same one is used by editors from a number of large publishers to detect plagiarism.

If a manuscript that is checked by one of these systems and found to be similar to work that is already published then the percentage similarity will be reported and the precise sources of the similarity will be provided in the output. The system can take into account reference lists and quotes in the text and is also capable of detecting similar runs of words and phrases that may remain after someone has tried to cover up their plagiarism. Clearly, the output from one of these programmes requires some interpretation by the editor and it is appreciated that zero percent similarity is unlikely to be achieved. The ethical and legal aspects of publication are covered in more detail in Chapter 12. Suffice to say here that as part of the editorial process detection of plagiarism of any kind can result in a number of serious outcomes for the author(s).

What action can be taken if plagiarism is detected?

If unethical practice is detected then the editor will investigate and most publishers adhere to the COPE guidelines, which they may link to their own web pages but which are freely available to authors and editors on the Internet (www.publicationethics.org; Accessed 15 May 2011). The COPE web page contains invaluable information and case studies but, in terms of investigative procedures and action it contains a series of algorithms the editor and the publisher can follow (see Chapter 12 for this algorithm). For example, if plagiarism is suspected then the editor is obliged to investigate and this will now be done using the plagiarism detection software mentioned previously.

If substantial similarity is detected then the publishers will be alerted and, depending on the publishers' own procedures, either the editor or the publisher will communicate with the author under investigation. Whatever malpractice is suspected, the corresponding author will be informed as to what has been detected, what the publisher's initial assessment of the situation is and the author asked to provide an explanation. The severity of subsequent action will depend on the response of the corresponding author and this may range from a frank admission, through some genuine misunderstanding or poor, rather than unethical practice, to stark denial either of any similarity or any wrongdoing.

Where there is an immediate admission of guilt then it is not uncommon for the manuscript to be withdrawn. This may be done prior to publication if the paper is still at the manuscript or proof stage; if the paper has already been published then a retraction statement will be published on the webpage and the paper, which usually remains on the webpage, watermarked with 'Retraction' on the Internet page of the journal but not of course in the already published paper-based version, and a notice posted in place of the paper or accompanying the paper to indicate that the contents were similar to other sources and with the agreement of the author(s) the paper had been withdrawn. Usually, no further action will be taken by the publishers.

However, where someone refuses to admit clearly unethical practice that has been unequivocally proven, then the paper will still be withdrawn but indicating that this action was taken by the publisher, and the author(s) will be reported to their institution, sometimes with serious consequences for their career.

Compiling issues of the journal

While most papers are accessed and read online these days and some journals exclusively publish online, hard copy issues are still compiled (that is articles are chosen for that issues by the editor) and are important for publicity purposes and are prominent on publishers' stands at conferences, for example. Compiled issues are also useful for producing special issues, which are sometimes sponsored by professional organisations and can then be bought and used for promotional purposes or included in conference packs.

Sometimes, these special issues are edited by guest editors – usually with the Editor-in-Chief having an oversight of the issue. Special issues may arise from conferences, where the papers are gathered into one issue, for example the special issue of *Nurse Education Today* that was co-published with *Nurse Education in Practice* following the inaugural NET/NEP 2006 1st International Nursing Education Conference in Vancouver, Canada (http://www.sciencedirect.com/science/journal/14715953/6; Accessed 23 April 2012). Alternatively, special issues may cluster around one specific theme, for example the regular special issues on Complementary and Alternative Medicines published in *Journal of Clinical Nursing*.

A recent development is the compilation of 'virtual' online issues whereby papers that have already been published are gathered in one online issue – usually made available free – and then used for promotional purposes (see previous reference to the *Journal of Clinical Nursing*: Violence Virtual Issue). In fact, there is no reason why special issues should be confined to one journal; special issues can also be compiled across cognate journals in the same publishing company.

Media exposure

Once papers are published, some editors and publishers select papers they think will be of particular interest from the media perspective. Usually these will be papers addressing topical issues or with particularly interesting findings. It can be hard to predict what will be of interest and specialist help from media consultants or journalists may be required. In addition, publishers set up systems to alert potential readers about journal content including email alerts of contents once they are published online and RSS feeds; readers need to register for these and they are always free. Journals are also using social networking sites to effect what is known as 'viral marketing' and World Wide Web links to contents alert. Journal contents and specific papers of interest are advertised using Twitter® or alerted on Facebook® or similar sites.

Conclusion

This chapter has hopefully given you a valuable insight into the publication process of an article you submit for possible publication in a journal of your choice. The role of the editor or Editor-in-Chief is critical to the quality of this process and also to ensuring both the quality of the scholarship and the standards of publication in any journal. They can be considered 'gatekeepers' of the scholarly community, ensuring that the knowledge translated and transferred through their journal internationally is of the highest ethical standards and through their leadership the editorial team becomes established as fair and supportive of any author who submits their work for consideration in their journals.

References

Hames, I. (2007) *Peer Review and Manuscript Management in Scientific Journals.* Oxford: Blackwell Publishing Ltd.
Miser, H.J. (1998) Journal editing as I see it. *CBE Views*, 22, 71-75.

Further reading

Ware, M. (2008) Peer Review: benefits, perceptions and alternatives. Publishing Research Consortium Summary Papers 4, *Publishing Research Consortium*, London.

Websites

Peer review in scientific publications: government and research councils UK responses to the committee's eight report of session 2010-12. Tenth special report of session 2010-12. Available at: http://www.publications.parliament .uk/pa/cm201012/cmselect/cmsctech/1535/1535.pdf [23 April 2012].

Chapter 11

Being a Journal Reviewer: Good Practice in Reviewing

Karen Holland

School of Nursing, Midwifery and Social Work, University of Salford, Salford, UK

Introduction

As an editor of a journal I am reliant on a team of volunteer reviewers who, in Emden's (1996) words, make a significant contribution to the scholarship of a discipline and the work of others; yet this is often an unacknowledged form of scholarship. If a journal is peer reviewed, that denotes that there is some kind of review process of its manuscripts prior to publication, and it is this role and what makes a good and effective reviewer that is the focus of this chapter.

I will establish what exactly is peer review, why individuals become reviewers, what criteria editors have for becoming a reviewer for a journal, how a reviewer carries out the role, how they give feedback to authors and the kind of comments that are acceptable for authors to be able to learn from and use effectively in the revision of their papers or to improve their paper, should it be rejected. These aspects of what it means to be a journal reviewer will be illustrated by examples and activities that new and established reviewers can learn from.

It is also possible to become a reviewer for book publishers, for book proposals submitted in draft. This can be very rewarding, and publishers rely on such experts to advise on whether or not a book is needed and, most importantly, commercially whether students and others will purchase the book (see Chapter 6). Some individuals can also be invited to review complete manuscripts of books, especially if they have already offered constructive feedback on the development of the initial book proposal. This can also be rewarding as you can see how the book has developed and the authors acted upon everyone's review comments as appropriate. The main purpose of this chapter,

Writing for Publication in Nursing and Healthcare: Getting It Right, First Edition.
Edited by Karen Holland and Roger Watson.
© 2012 John Wiley & Sons, Ltd. Published 2012 by John Wiley & Sons, Ltd.

however, is to focus on reviewing for a journal and the role of the reviewer of journal articles.

What is peer review?

A research report (Ware, 2008) commissioned by the Publishers Research Consortium focused entirely on 'peer review, its benefits and perception alternatives'. This report is a fascinating insight into the world of peer review and the role of journals and a link to the website where you can download the report can be found at the end of this chapter.

The report cites that:

> [P]eer review is the process of subjecting an author's scholarly manuscript to the scrutiny of others who are experts in the same field, prior to publication in the journal.
>
> (Ware, 2008, p. 4)

This notion of scrutiny of a paper is also noted by Molassiotis and Richardson (2004) who offer helpful editorial advice to readers and potential authors of the European Journal of Oncology Nursing.

As an editor, the role of the reviewer is critical in the decision-making role, about which papers to publish and why; therefore, choosing reviewers for specific journals is essential to ensure a high-quality publication and for authors to know that their papers are being reviewed by someone who understands their work and who will give them constructive advice with regard to their work.

Types of peer review

Before we look at selecting reviewers and why you may wish to consider becoming one, it is worth considering the systems associated with peer review.

There are three types of reviews:

(1) Single-blinded review
(2) Double-blinded reviews
(3) Open reviews

Single-blinded review is where the author's identity is known to the reviewer but that the reviewer's identity is hidden from the author (Ware, 2008). Double-blinded peer review is where neither author nor reviewer know each other's identity and it has benefits, in that unlike single-blinded review where there could be the potential for bias, it offers the opposite.

Open review is where both authors and reviewer's identities are known to each other and in some cases are published together. It is, according to advocates of the system, a much fairer system:

... because they argue, somebody making an important judgement on the work of others should not do so in secret and that reviewers will produce better work and avoid offhand, careless or rude comments when their identity is known.

(Ware, 2008, p. 6)

Many nursing and healthcare-related journals use either single- or double-blinded peer review, the latter being the most prevalent. Whatever system is used, the ultimate responsibility for whether a paper gets published or not resides with the editor and the editor's role is covered in Chapter 10.

The role of a reviewer

Whatever the system of review, there are specific responsibilities in the role of a reviewer. These are important if you are considering the role. To illustrate some of the responsibilities of being a reviewer as well as the kind of criteria that editors may look for in accepting an application to become a journal reviewer I draw on personal experience as an editor and being a reviewer for several journals. Each journal has its own criteria for acceptance onto a panel of reviewers (some journal links are found at the end of this chapter) but there are basic criteria that are applicable to all.

What do we look for in a reviewer?

(1) For *Nurse Education in Practice* (*NEP*) journal you need to be knowledgeable about nurse education generally and able to offer specialist knowledge in an area such as assessment, teaching and learning strategies, new technology in learning, clinical simulation and learning in practice (for examples of types of articles published in the journal that reflect these topics see http://www.elsevier.com/wps/find/journaldescription .cws_home/623062/description#description).

For more practice-focused journals such as *Journal of Clinical Nursing* (*JCN*) (for access to published articles that reflect the breadth of specialist topic areas see http://www.blackwellpublishing.com/journal.asp? ref=0962-1067).

(2) NEP journal also looks for some subject specialist knowledge – either in relation to a field of practice such as mental health, health promotion and critical care, or in aspects of research, especially the conduct of research and the methodologies used. Most reviewers have experience of both of these and we require every applicant to complete a reviewer expertise form, which enables me as editor to access the right person for the

review. For other journals such as *Nursing in Critical Care* (http://www
.wiley.com/bw/journal.asp?ref=1362-1017) or *Intensive and Critical Care
Nursing* (http://www.elsevier.com/wps/find/journaldescription.cws_home
/623043/description#description) there is an expectation that the reviewer has expertise is the field of critical and/or intensive care as an
essential requirement. Most journals now have support for reviewer
websites where you can download information on reviewing and related
activities (e.g. see http://www.elsevier.com/wps/find/reviewershome
.reviewers/reviewersguidelines). However, in the area of methodologies,
for example, some reviewers are not nurses or educators but are from
other disciplines. On NEP, for example, there are librarians, statisticians
and information scientists who give a valued contribution to the review
process and, as Pierson (2011, p. 3) indicated, reviewers are selected
based on their expertise relevant to the content of the manuscript. This
advice can be found in the excellent publication produced by *Nurse,
Author & Editor* for Wiley-Blackwell who have excellent resources for
authors, reviewers and editors (for reviewers support resources see
http://www.nurseauthoreditor.com/forreviewers.asp).

(3) It is preferable for a reviewer to have some personal publishing experience,
but this is not a compulsory requirement for all journals. As an editor I
choose a combination of different experiences in reviewers and often new
reviewers are matched with more experienced ones. It is also important
to give feedback to new reviewers to ensure they continue to undertake
the role and develop their skills as part of their professional development.

(4) It is essential that reviewers have a commitment to promoting scholarship,
as the feedback they give is not only evidence of their own scholarly
contribution (Emden, 1996) but also their contribution to the scholarship
of others and therefore, the scholarship of the wider discipline.

(5) Editors are responsible for ensuring that a reviewer has the requisite skills
and knowledge to give constructive feedback not only to authors but also
to editors who have the decision-making responsibility of whether to reject
a paper or ask for revision. Editors also have responsibility for making
the initial review of articles submitted to ensure that reviewer's time is
not wasted in reviewing articles that would need significant revision or
possibly have been sent in to the wrong journal in the first place (see
Chapter 11 for editorial process).

What do we expect from reviewers?

Reviewers are expected to provide editors with timely and appropriate comments on an author's submission. Timely means there will be set minimum time
limits for reviewers to return their reviews and when that deadline passes they
normally receive a reminder, periodically. In some journals like NEP if there
is no response after a set time the reviewer is 'un-invited' from the review
process of the paper to ensure a timely response to authors on their work.

This does not always happen, but most of the time it works as the editor will have assigned more than two reviewers to the process.

Very efficient electronic submission and process management tools exist that enable editors to identify at least two main reviewers and also two alternative reviewers, to ensure that there is continuity of reviewers. Key expectations in addition to the aforementioned are given in the following text.

To be constructive in their comments to authors

This is possibly the most important aspect of what we expect from reviewers after making a decision for the editor on whether to accept or reject an article or ask the author(s) to make revisions. The feedback should follow what has been asked for by the journal guide for reviewers or the template used for electronic submission of the review (e.g. see Boxes 11.1 and 11.2).

The reviewer is asked to comment on various aspects of the article – much like giving feedback and marking of a student's assignment – the same principles apply, and for those wishing to review but who think they do not have the skills, if you are good at marking and giving constructive feedback to students and have received positive feedback yourself about this then you have the skills.

Regardless of the type of feedback requested, it needs to be constructive. Let us look at some examples using Pierson's (2011) framework as a guide (additional ones can be found in Pierson (2011) guidance for reviewers) (Table 11.1). The examples cited here are all from real reviewer comments I have seen as an editor, although some of these have been combined to illustrate what

Box 11.1   Reviewer guidance (general principles of good practice)

- Read the article first to get a general overview of its content.
- Undertake a more detailed reading of the article to determine if it is easy to understand.
- Consider all aspects of the message the author(s) are trying to convey.
- Does the author use a large number of abbreviations and/or acronyms that detract from reading the article?
- Is it possible to discern whether the author's first language is not English?
- Is the grammar and structure of the article in keeping with what you would expect from an author submitting a paper to an international peer-reviewed journal?
- Is the referencing style in keeping with the author guidelines?
- Has the author followed the author guidelines for submission of the paper?

Box 11.2 Reviewer guide for *Nurse Education in Practice* (NEP) – key issues

Specific reviewer comments for the author

Does the article:
 (1) Meet the aims and scope of NEP? Yes/No
 Comments:

 (2) Adhere to the recommended format for journal articles? Yes/No
 Comments:

 (3) Exceed the recommended word limit? Yes/No
 Comments:

 (4) Are the aims of the article clearly stated? Yes/No
 Comments:

 (5) Is the cited literature relevant and reflect current views? Yes/No
 Comments:

 (6) Provide a new perspective/innovation in nurse education practice
 and/or healthcare education generally? Yes/No
 Comments:

 (7) Provide an understanding of its content and/or applicability for an
 international readership? Yes/No
 Comments:

For research papers

 (8) Does the article outline the research design, including methodologies and methods that are well justified? Yes/No
 Comments:

 (9) Are access/ethical issues discussed? Yes/No
 Comments:

 (10) Are data analysis/findings clearly indicated and discussed? Yes/No
 Comments:

 (11) Is the statistical data (if any) accurate/clearly represented? If you
 are not comfortable reviewing stats please advise. Yes/No
 Comments:
 ....

Overall comments on the paper
Here the reviewer makes an overall judgement on the article that is supported by comments in each of the relevant categories, including possible confidential comments to the editor on issues such as suspected plagiarism, which the editor will need to investigate.

Recommendations
Due to electronic submission of articles and reviewer decisions, the categories open to the editor has now been expanded to take account of a range of feedback options, which has improved the editor's communication with authors. Reviewers are asked in the review, however, to make an initial judgement on the main categories of either revision: minor or major with reconsideration by the reviewer; more suitable for publication in another journal or reject and not suitable for publication in the journal. These comments are supported by detailed feedback to authors together with comments in each of the essential categories required.

kind of comments reviewers make for author feedback. You will note that there are two in relation to plagiarism issues, which is unfortunately becoming more prevalent across all disciplines (see Chapter 12).

What are the basic and specific guidelines the reviewer may use in the review of an article?

As you can see from Table 11.1 there are key issues that reviewers are required to consider when reviewing articles and how reviewers are meant to respond to in terms of feedback to authors.

In Box 11.1 you can see the general principles of good practice in reviewing any article and in Box 11.2 the more specific requirements you may be required to complete by the editor. The one illustrated here is from NEP. It is anticipated that any reviewer would adopt the basic principles of review in addition to the more specific guidelines of the journal itself.

Activity 1

(1) Identify a journal that you believe you could review for. See if there are any call for reviewers in the online pages, and if you think you can do this then apply using the guidance provided.

(2) Pick out a random paper from a journal you are familiar with and read regularly. Imagine you are seeing this for the first time as a reviewer and undertake a review using some agreed guidance (a template is seen in Box 11.1 and a specific reviewer one in Box 11.2).

Table 11.1 Examples of feedback.

Areas for feedback (general)	Unhelpful comments	Constructive comments
Aims of the article	Unclear	The aims of the article do not appear to reflect what the author has written about and also is not reflected in the title of the article. Recommend that they re-visit the aims again and consider amending the title.
The literature used in the article	Not very good. Many dated references, which do not add anything to the evidence.	Although the author has used supporting evidence, they have not undertaken account of more recent literature available on the topic (see examples). While the references used are still valid, they need to demonstrate the additional up to date ones as well to show that they are using best evidence in their study.
Grammar and typographical issues	This is appalling throughout and authors need to consider use of English language in future papers.	It is apparent that the author's first language is not English due to grammar and sentence construction. I would advise that they seek advice from someone who has first language English or who has published in international English language journals previously. The basis of the article is good with potential for publication. The typo's in the paper are, however, not acceptable and the author needs to have the paper proof read before any re-submission.
Research methodology, methods and data analysis	The author clearly has not used phenomenology and not sure that they completely understand it in relation to the methods used and subsequent analysis.	There are major issues with the research design section of this paper. The author states that the methodology was phenomenology and reflected the experience of the key participants. However, they appear to have used a short survey of some kind with open-ended questions to which they have analysed using narrative analysis and state that this reflected the experience of the participants in relation to the questions asked. This is confusing and does not meet the standard required for the journal as it impacts on the findings and the subsequent discussion and recommendations. On this basis, the article does not meet the journal's expectations.

(continued)

Table 11.1 (*Continued*)

Areas for feedback (general)	Unhelpful comments	Constructive comments
Ethical issues	None at all noted.	The author does not mention any ethical issues in the research section of the article, although does indicate that participants could opt out of the study if they wished to. As this article focused on interview of service users, this is of some concern that no ethical approval appears to have been given. It may of course be an oversight on behalf of the author in writing up the article, but they need to inform the editor that approval had been given before any further decision is made. It is essential that in any article involving participants, whether students or service users, some reference is made to request for ethical approval or advice from an ethics committee to determine if it is required.
Evidence of any plagiarism (1)	None that I can see although not entirely familiar with all the literature in this field.	Using the journal check system for plagiarism it is evident that there is some self -plagiarism from another published paper linked to this study. On comparing both papers there is a large part of the literature review that has been used in this paper from the previously published one. This is not good practice and the author needs to take cognisance of this for any future publications. It may of course be a simple misunderstanding of the protocols for publishing from same study.
Evidence of any plagiarism (2)	The author has plagiarised sections from a paper I wrote in 2006! and also sections from another author in the same field but passing it off as their own! Unbelievable bad practice.	On reading the paper I was drawn to key aspects of the literature review and also aspects of the discussion section and thought that it looked familiar. The actual paragraphs in question were from a paper I had previously published on this subject in 2006. On further reading it became clear that there were other sections that were not attributed to anyone, which were directly lifted from another colleague's published work and assumed to have been the author's own work. This was clearly not evidence of any confusion in publishing protocols and the author needs to be advised of the seriousness of the situation and a decision made as to any further work being considered for publication in this journal. I realise that this places the editor in a difficult position.

Source: Based on Pierson (2011), p. 6.

Be willing to help authors develop their papers for publication

Reviewers need to be prepared to offer their experience and expertise, together with a willingness to help authors develop their paper for publication. We can see from the examples in Table 11.1 that there is a difference between one reviewer and another who is prepared to offer constructive advice to authors. New authors are particularly grateful for this supportive approach, even if their paper is rejected. Editors have a responsibility to monitor very negative and unhelpful reviewer comments and, if necessary, to modify or add to in order to help the author. It is also editors' responsibility to communicate with reviewers to give them feedback about the quality of their reviews. Although it is appreciated that this is a voluntary role, in agreeing to become a member of a panel of reviewers there is an expectation of good feedback to help authors and, of course, by doing so add value to the scholarship of the discipline.

Advise editors on the overall quality of the papers they review

In either accepting an invitation to review for a journal (and new systems enable editors to access potential reviewers through linked databases, such as SCOPUS in Elsevier journals) or responding to a call for reviewers and being accepted, it is taken for granted that advising the editor on the overall quality of an article as well as key aspects of it as highlighted in Table 11.1 is essential for the editor to make a decision about the manuscript. This becomes even more important when two reviewers in a double-blinded peer-review system have very opposing views about the quality of the article for publication in a specific journal. Obviously, if there are comments on plagiarism then this overrides the main comments due to the potential damage to the journal itself in terms of its reputation and also any outcome for the author concerned.

Keep to deadlines for return of reviewed papers

When reviewers accept the role they will normally be given some kind of induction to the journal with regard to time for reviewing an article. It is usually specified in the letter of invitation to review the article and also advice on what to do should they be unable to meet this deadline or wish their name to be suspended from reviewing for a period. It is important to advise the editorial office and editor as soon as possible if this is the situation. Reasons vary from family bereavement, hospitalisation, holidays, periods of sabbaticals or pressure of work.

Meeting deadlines is important if the journal is to retain a reputation for short turnaround in decisions about articles. There are periods from personal experience when the deadlines have to be extended and authors who inquire are made aware of this. This often occurs from about middle of July to middle of September, mainly due to reviewers and editorial team members taking their holidays or having sabbaticals to undertake extended study or research. The main issue is keeping editors informed as much as possible about change in circumstances so that they do not add to any pressure or distress by sending electronic pre-organised messages. However, if reviewers persistently refuse to carry out reviews they are normally removed from the panel of reviewers.

Keep up to date with what is happening in nursing

This requirement for becoming a reviewer might seem like common sense. However, it becomes apparent that when reviewers send back their comments, even though in general they are very positive, that one area where advice to authors is of value is how their article fits in to the bigger picture of what is either happening in their discipline or whether they have taken account of the author's understanding of the international context. In reviewing for an international journal this is an essential requirement and, from personal experience, having to consider the wider context has meant reading around subjects and adding to one's own body of knowledge about the topic being reviewed and how it applies in other countries worldwide. It is astounding how 'ethnocentric' authors are, however, in how they view the world around them in relation to making their articles either easily understood by readers in other countries or including literature from outside their own country in the evidence base to their articles. Of course, this is not always a requirement but the authors need to make clear to readers what they are talking about and of course explaining the dreaded abbreviations and acronyms! Reviewers will pick up on these and this could make a difference to whether or not they recommend acceptance, revisions or rejections.

Reviewing for an international nursing education/practice journal: additional issues

Take into account an author's writing in English as a second language

As mentioned, it is essential that reviewers recognise whether or not English is the first language of the author. It is often easy to see this, as the author will identify the country the study may have been carried out in, but this is not always apparent. Of course, it could be that the author has just written a paper that includes poor sentence construction, grammar and lack of care. This latter paper may have already been reviewed on submission by the editor and rejected prior to review with advice to the author on future quality of their submission to that or any other journal. If it is obvious the author's first language is not English then guidance can be offered as to how to improve this and many journals now have additional services that can be accessed to help authors with this aspect of their written work. It is essential that this is conveyed in a sensitive manner to the authors, either by the reviewer or by the editor. Most authors will welcome this additional support. Obviously, if the paper as a whole is not acceptable because the English is so poor that it would take major revision and extended time to develop, the author is advised of this and normally rejected. If there is potentially new insight into a field of practice that can be discerned, for example from evidence presented, then an editor may recommend that they withdraw the paper at this time and consider the reviewer comments, find assistance in re-drafting their paper and re-submitting as a new submission in the future. This is not a complete rejection of the paper but offers an opening for an author who is serious about publishing their work to work on their article without the additional pressure of deadlines. It also encourages authors to write in international journals where English is the main medium of communication and adds to the evidence base of a discipline, as well encouraging transnational communication.

Applicability of papers for different international and cultural contexts

Aspects of this have already been noted, such as not being 'ethnocentric' in writing an article and explaining the context surrounding the topic of the article, an example is the continual reference to the NMC or the NHS or SHA's without thinking if someone reading the article in another country will know what these are or the documents referenced with them if no context to their use has been made. Reviewers need to ensure that the editor is made aware of this but in many instances if this is a major issue, the article can often be rejected prior to review. Many journals have an increasing number of manuscripts being submitted and competition for publication is increasing. All journals are allocated a page budget for their papers if they have both electronic and paper-based versions. Of course, open access journals and other new online only journals may have a different model of working, but even here the quality of the publications are still important and they also have various peer-review systems that adopt similar structures to those discussed here.

Some of the issues in this chapter clearly have messages for reviewers or potential reviewers about their own writing for publication journeys; reviewing for a journal also helps the reviewer identify with issues they had not considered in their own endeavour to write for publication.

What the editor and publisher can do for the reviewer?

Reviewing for a journal is not a one-way process. Editors and publishers also have a responsibility to reviewers; without them there would not be peer review and despite the discussions about the value of open access journals and their peer-review systems as well as the ability of academics working in universities to be able to upload work that may not have been peer reviewed internally, Ware (2008, p. 4) highlights that:

peer review is widely supported by academics, who overwhelmingly (93%) disagreed in our greatly helps scientific communication and believed (83%) that without peer review there would be no control.

This finding is based on respondents from the Thomson Scientific database and the number of respondents who could respond to all questions related to peer review was 3040 and the number of editors who responded to their questions was 632 – the respondents were from all subject areas and disciplines –from science journals and arts and humanities as well as medical and nursing journals.

The editor should be prepared to give feedback on the skills and contribution of the reviewer to both the authors and to the overall quality of the journal's publications. Many journals announce annually the names of all those reviewers who have reviewed papers for them in the previous 12 months and this is valuable in terms of demonstrating to their peers and managers that they are making a contribution to the scholarly community as a whole in their discipline and subject specialist field.

The publisher can also contribute to the value of the reviewer in the publishing process. Although financial remuneration is not an option for most journals, often the publisher will enable other options for reviewers such as a reduction in cost of journal subscription, access to other resources within the review process such as access to online abstracts, publications and other material to help in the review process as well as for their own scholarly use.

Some reviewers who have made significant contribution to the journal's peer-review process can be invited to become members of international advisory or editorial boards. This is of added value where this kind of 'academic presence' is important to their careers.

Why become a reviewer?

There are three main reasons that we can consider for becoming a reviewer, some of which I have alluded to in previous sections. These are:

(1) Personal and professional development.
(2) Keeping abreast of developments in nurse education.
(3) Contributing to scholarship of others.

We can consider these in turn.

Personal and professional development

The reviewer may apply to become a reviewer in response to a call for reviewers or be invited via an integral system to the review process; they may have been recommended by a reviewer who is unable to review at the time required or who may suggest that the person nominated has more expertise in the focus of the article. This may be a personal choice on behalf of the individual in terms of their own personal development or may be something they have discussed with a mentor or as part of their ongoing professional development.

Keeping abreast of developments in nurse education/nursing practice/research

When discussing with reviewers during writing for publication workshops, some reviewers state that reviewing not only helps them with their own writing skills, but in reading and reviewing articles regularly it also enables them to keep abreast of developments in a specific field or topic, which subsequently supports their evidence-based teaching.

Contributing to scholarship of others

For many, this is possibly a more altruistic reason for becoming a reviewer. For many, it is a genuine decision that extends from their own work and supporting others. Being a reviewer is a key role for editors and publishers, including being essential to the quality of what a journal publishes but also to its reputation in the academic and publishing fields. Reviewers are in essence the gatekeepers to quality evidence-based publications as well as offering their expertise to assist in the development of authors and their work.

Summary

Becoming and being a reviewer is a key role in writing for publication practice. It is as Emden (1996) states also 'an act of scholarship'. It is important that not only those who work in a higher education environment consider becoming a reviewer but also experienced practitioners who have specialist knowledge and skills relevant to the field in which authors submit their articles to either a generalist or specialist journal. I would like to end with the same quote I used in my editorial on the peer-review process (Holland, 2002, p. 71) from Emden's paper, where she states that:

> Hardy (1991) states that 'accepting the role of reviewer means prestige is being conferred upon you'. It is timely, therefore, as nursing journals proudly declare their peer-reviewed status, that those who participate in the process acknowledge the scholarly significance of their work. By openly articulating the nature or unique style of our work, we might also experience the benefits of a peer-review process.

References

Emden, C. (1996) Manuscript reviewing: too long a concealed form of scholarship? *Nursing Inquiry*, 3, 195–199.

Hardy, L.K. (1991) Peer review and accountability. *The Canadian Journal of Nursing Research*, 23, 3–5.

Holland, K. (2002) Reviewing papers and the peer review process (Editorial). *Nurse Education in Practice*, 2, 71.

Molassiotis, A. & Richardson, A. (2004) The peer review process in an academic journal. *European Oncology Nursing Society*, 8, 359–362.

Pierson, C. (2011) *Reviewing Journal Manuscripts*. Oxford: Wiley-Blackwell.

Ware, M. (2008) Peer review: benefits, perceptions and alternatives. Publishing Research Consortium Summary Papers 4, Publishing Research Consortium, London. Available at: http://www.publications.parliament.uk/pa/cm201012/cmselect/cmsctech/1535/1535.pdf [Accessed 9 June 2012].

Further reading

Happell, B. (2011) Responding to reviewers' comments as part of writing for publication. *Nurse Researcher*, 18(4), 23–27.

Rosenbaum, P. (2002) In my opinion: reflections of a journal reviewer. *Child: Care, Health & Development*, 28(4), 331–333.

Websites

This is a link to the Journal of Nursing Scholarship website, which is part of Sigma Theta Tau International Honor Society of Nursing publications. Available at: http://www.nursingsociety.org/Publications/Journals/Pages/JNSReviewer.aspx [Accessed 23 April 2012].

This is a link to the Nurse Researcher RCN publication website, which subscribers to the journal can access directly, and also has information on various activities, sample research papers and other links to online resources and RCN journals. Available at: http://nurseresearcher.rcnpublishing.co.uk/ [Accessed 23 April 2012].

The Nurse Author & Editor website for authors, editors and reviewers and edited by one of our chapter editors, Dr Charon Pierson. Available at: http://www.nurseauthoreditor.com/ [Accessed 7 October 2011].

The links to Elsevier publication websites information for authors. Available at: http://www.elsevier.com/wps/find/authorsview.authors/landing_main [Accessed 23 April 2012] and http://www.nursingplus.com/ [Accessed 23 April 2012] (also has additional resource links to Nurse, Author & Editor material).

Chapter 12

Ethical and Legal Aspects of Publishing: Avoiding Plagiarism and Other Issues

Charon A. Pierson

Center for Aging, University of Texas, El Paso, TX, USA

Introduction

The pillars of ethical reasoning that support the conduct and dissemination of nursing research extend to the arena of publishing. Practical rules have evolved to prohibit plagiarism, fabrication of data or any behaviour that stems from competing interests. This chapter addresses many of the common ethical problems faced by authors, reviewers and editors with a case study and discussion/resolution of the issues involved. Resources for authors, reviewers and editors are provided as appropriate. We begin, however, with some background on recent events that have brought the dilemma of ethics in publishing to the forefront.

Dilemma of ethics in publishing

As clinicians, researchers, academics and consumers of healthcare we make the assumption that what we read in peer-reviewed publications is true or at least verifiable. We base our practice decisions and develop new research based on the findings of other researchers. When that base, the foundation, is tainted, that which follows becomes suspect. The case of Poehlman (Sox and Rennie, 2006) illustrates the ripple effect of scientific misconduct. Dr. Poehlman's research and publication record came under scrutiny and was thoroughly investigated by the Office of Research Integrity (ORI) (2000) and his university with the resulting finding of publication of fabricated research in ten different articles in ten different journals.

Writing for Publication in Nursing and Healthcare: Getting It Right, First Edition.
Edited by Karen Holland and Roger Watson.
© 2012 John Wiley & Sons, Ltd. Published 2012 by John Wiley & Sons, Ltd.

It is a basic assumption that all works in circulation written by an author who has committed scientific misconduct such as plagiarism or fabrication should be considered suspect until proven otherwise (Committee on Publication Ethics (COPE), www.publicationethics.org). In the case of Dr. Poehlman, at the time of the decision of the ORI, 186 of his publications were listed in the Science Citation Index Database (Thompson Science, Philadelphia, PA); these 186 papers had accrued a total of 3007 citations (Sox and Rennie, 2006). This means that a possible 3007 studies, reviews, opinions, case studies or other publications have based some degree of conclusion or provided some degree of support for new ideas, treatments or interventions based upon a possibly flawed foundation.

There are many other cases of widespread contamination of the scientific record such as Dr. Wakefield's biased research linking autism to the measles, mumps, rubella vaccine (Godlee, 2011) and Dr. Reuben's falsified data on COX2 inhibitors that changed the way pain medicine was practiced in the United States (Borrell, 2009). The degree of harm caused by scientific misconduct of these researchers is difficult to quantify; some of the outcomes are just beginning to unfold.

Recent research has estimated that the harm to patients from scientific misconduct can be significant. Steen (2011a) reported that one primary research paper retracted because of fraud might have jeopardised the surgical pain management in as many as 7076 patients subsequently enrolled in similar studies. The list of retracted articles on the US National Library of Medicine (www.ncbi.nlm.nih.gov/pubmed; Accessed 5 November 2011) revealed 1937 retracted articles, some of which were from nursing journals. It is not clear which of these retracted articles has potential to cause harm to humans and which are retracted for duplicate publication, plagiarism or data fabrication. Most of the sensational cases from recent history, however, seem to contain some element of conflict of interest (COI) on the part of researchers receiving money and gifts from drug and device manufacturers. The issue of COI or competing interests is a good starting point to illustrate ethical dilemmas in writing, reviewing, conducting and publishing research.

Conflict of interest or competing interests

The purpose of any peer-reviewed scientific publication is the dissemination of cutting-edge, unbiased, well-written information, whether that is research, reviews, case studies, editorials or any other form of communication. COIs pose a threat to that goal, with Lo and Field (2009) stating:

A conflict of interest is a set of circumstances that creates a risk that professional judgment or actions regarding a primary interest will be unduly influenced by a secondary interest.

(Lo and Field, 2009, p. 46)

Authors, reviewers and editors must understand what might constitute primary and secondary interests in order to maintain transparency regarding potential competing interests. Financial enrichment, strongly held beliefs, career advancement or image enhancement can be powerful secondary interests that drive participation in authorship, research and publishing. To determine if secondary interests exist, editors request disclosure of any secondary interests, particularly financial relationships with companies that manufacture drugs, devices or clinical tests. The International Council of Medical Journal Editors (ICMJE) has developed an electronic form that includes disclosure information specific to biomedical manuscripts from conception through submission (ICMJE uniform disclosure form for potential COIs, www.icmje.org).

The purpose of the form is to provide editors with basic information about potential competing interests related to a submitted manuscript or review. There is no intent to establish if undue influence occurred; however, a reasonable person examining the form should be able to determine if the appearance of possible influence is sufficient to warrant additional query.

The crucial piece of information, whether or not undue influence occurred, cannot be answered. What can be answered is whether the situation creates an appearance of undue influence, in which case, complete disclosure should accompany the manuscript for review and publication. In the case study that follows, decide what information is pertinent to disclosure for a nurse submitting a manuscript to a peer-reviewed journal.

Case study 1   Potential conflicts of interest

An experienced wound care nurse conducts a clinical trial of a new wound dressing (a biologic compound embedded in the dressing) sponsored by company Z. The nurse receives an all-expense-paid trip to a resort area for training in the new dressing research protocol and all expenses for the clinical trial are covered via payments to the practice where she works. All data are managed by company Z and the nurse receives only a final analysis summary. Company Z hires company A, a communications company, to write a manuscript for submission to a peer-reviewed journal and to prepare a poster for presentation at an important international meeting. The nurse is listed as sole author. Company Z also puts the nurse on their speaker bureau and provides her with slides to do presentations around the country, paying all her expenses. At the time of submission of the manuscript, the nurse's boss, Dr. B, demands to be second author on the article without having done anything other than reading the final manuscript.

Ghosts, guests and sponsors

Issues arising from the above case study include *ghost writing*, *guest authorship* and *sponsorship of presenters*. Whether or not a COI has occurred on the part of the nurse depends on how the nurse handled the various issues in this scenario.

Sponsorship of clinical trials is not uncommon in the medical community. Institutions that receive US government support for research must adhere to guidelines promulgated by the ORI (2000) and similar requirements are in place in other locations such as the UK Research Integrity Office (http://www.ukrio.org/home), an independent advisory body that provides guidance on how to address fraud and misconduct in research. Registration of clinical trials is governed by countries or regions, although, many international trials register at the National Institutes of Health ClinicalTrials.gov website.

The first question that arises in the case study is, 'was the clinical trial registered as required?' Certain requirements of trial registration help ensure that ethical protocols are in place and followed. The fact that the nurse was paid to attend training should be disclosed but is a reasonable covered expense. The drug and device industry has come under scrutiny about training programs and investigator meetings, but journal editors are not the enforcers of any regulations for that industry.

Ghost writing has been exposed in medical publications in recent years (US Senate Committee on Finance, 2010) and is expressly prohibited by many journals. Ghost-written articles are crafted by professional medical writers hired by pharmaceutical or communications companies and presented as submissions by professionals such as nurses or physicians without acknowledgement of the writing assistance of the professional writer. Traditionally, this has been more a problem for medical journals, but nursing journals have not escaped scrutiny.

The rationale for submitting a ghost-written manuscript from a prominent professional is to improve the credibility of the work and the likelihood of acceptance. Professional writing assistance can have a legitimate role in developing manuscripts; however, the extent of involvement and any financial support must be completely disclosed at the time of submission. The term ghost writing could apply to the nurse in this case if writing assistance from a writer hired by company A is not acknowledged in the manuscript. Guidance on the role of publications professionals (e.g. writers, editors and publication managers) is available from the American Medical Writers Association (www.amwa.org), and from the revised *Good Publication Practices* document available online (GPP-2 guidelines; www.gpp-guidelines.org).

The ICMJE uniform disclosure form should accompany any submission in which funding and/or writing assistance has occurred. Transparency in funding, development and writing assistance are essential to eliminating ghost writing. One might also question the legitimacy of the nurse as author because the data were controlled by the company and not her as the investigator. The GPP-2 guidelines urge that sponsors provide all investigators with complete access to the raw data, not the analysed and summarised version done by the sponsor.

Guest authorship is another potential problem in the case described. The guest author is Dr. B who has made no apparent contribution to the research or writing of the manuscript. The ICMJE defines an author as someone who has made a substantial contribution to the (1) conception, design or data acquisition, analysis or interpretation; (2) drafting or revising the manuscript for 'critical intellectual content' and (3) final approval of the manuscript (http://www.icmje.org/ethical_1author.html). Authors must meet all three conditions, the test of which is the ability to publicly defend all content within the manuscript. Previous cases in which sponsoring companies recruited well-known professionals to sign on as 'authors' of ghost-written manuscripts were the subject of the Grassley hearings (US Senate Committee on Finance, 2010) and resulted in significant changes in policies among industry leaders.

Other cases of competing interests

Authors are not the only ones subject to potential COI. Competing interests of reviewers and editors can influence the outcome of peer review and affect the literature of the discipline. Editorial policies at most journals reflect some 'bias screening' (Scott-Lichter et al., 2009) before assignment of reviewers. Some examples include policies requesting that reviewers declare potential financial, academic or intellectual conflicts that might preclude a fair and unbiased review. One journal that is seen to adopt good practice in this issue is the *Journal of Nursing Education,* where papers published all have a declaration statement that: 'The author has no financial or proprietary interest in the materials presented herein' (e.g. O'Neill, 2011).

Editors might have policies against soliciting reviewers who are from the same state or the same institution, or someone who is a known competitor of the author. Reviewers might be asked to sign COI disclosures for some journals. Bias in completed reviews might be detected by editors or authors, and in such cases, journal policies for appeal of a decision should be followed. Unfortunately, there is no foolproof way to prevent bias from competing interests; editors rely on the honesty of reviewers to comply with ethical standards. Cases of reviewer misconduct should be investigated by editors and reviewer policies should clearly state what is expected of reviewers. The next case illustrates a case from the COPE Council related to reviewer misconduct and COI.

Case study 2   Reviewer misconduct

COPE case 05-02 (http://www.publicationethics.org/case/reviewerauthor-conflict-interest) illustrates a COI on the part of a reviewer.

Dr. A accepted an invitation to review a newly submitted article within his area of expertise. He failed to complete the review within the allotted time frame and in the interim submitted an article on the same topic to the same journal that had asked for his review. The editors realised that there was significant overlap with the content of Dr. A's article and the article he had agreed but failed to review and asked for advice on what sanctions if any should derive from the incident. The COPE Council, among other things, advised the editors to review their cover letter to reviewers to specifically remind them that competing interests must be declared, particularly if the reviewer is working on something similar.

The conduct of Dr. A appeared to be unethical based on his failure to complete the review (The PLoS Medicine Editors, 2009) and his submission of a competing article to the same journal, although there was no accusation of plagiarism. He should have declared a COI stating that he was working on a very similar project and planned to submit his manuscript in the very near future to the same journal.

The aforementioned case illustrates another ethical issue for reviewers - *confidentiality*. All manuscripts should be treated confidentially; this means that reviewers should not discuss the manuscript with anyone else without permission of the editor. Reviewers should not make copies of manuscripts to use as references for their own work, for example copying the reference list to enhance the reviewer's own work or selecting portions of the reviewed manuscript to use in forthcoming manuscripts. Sharing of any reviews is at the discretion of the editor, and policies and procedures should be in place to assure that sharing is appropriate. For example when a manuscript is re-submitted after revisions, the reviews of the initial submission might be shared with subsequent reviewers for the purpose of clarifying any revisions made.

Reviewing manuscripts is difficult and time-consuming work that is mostly performed by peer volunteers. Reviewers have ethical obligations to report any competing interests, to perform their reviews in a timely manner, to provide constructive and respectful feedback to authors and to treat the content of the manuscript as privileged information. Most reviewers, authors and editors agree that the peer-review system is subjective and fraught with ethical dilemmas, yet it remains the dominant system for monitoring the scientific literature (Sieber, 2006; Scott-Lichter et al., 2009).

Research misconduct

Research misconduct is broadly defined as 'behaviour by a researcher, intentional or not, that falls short of good ethical and scientific standard' (Scott-Lichter et al., 2009, p. 38). In general terms, actions that are included in this definition include: unethical treatment of research subjects (human or animal), fabrication or falsification of data and plagiarism.

One of the most famous research projects in the United States, the Tuskegee Study, caused a change in research practices to protect human subjects; the law was the National Research Act of 1974. A serious ethical breach of deceiving human research subjects and withholding treatment of syphilis was committed by the US Public Health Service for 40 years (1932–1972) in order to monitor the natural history of syphilis among Black men from Tuskegee Alabama. Even after penicillin became the standard for treating syphilis, the Tuskegee subjects were prevented from obtaining treatment in the interest of preserving the scientific integrity of the study (for a timeline and extensive coverage of this subject see http://www.cdc.gov/tuskegee/index.html; Accessed 7 December 2011).

Reforms that occurred following the investigation into Tuskegee are outlined in the Belmont Report (1979) and led to the establishment of institutional review boards (IRBs), informed consent laws and better protection of all human subjects in the United States (an historical record of the Belmont Report can be found at http://www.hhs.gov/ohrp/archive/belmontArchive.html; Accessed 7 December 2011).

The original Declaration of Helsinki adopted by the World Medical Association in 1964 described the rights of individuals to make informed decisions regarding participation in research, and the first revision in 1975 reflected the concepts of IRBs (or ethical review boards) being established in the United States and other countries. Researchers must make a statement in their manuscripts about procedures in place to assure the protection of human subjects or the ethical treatment of animals. Failure to have such procedures in place or failure to include adequate explanation of those protections in a manuscript will likely result in rejection of the paper, and possibly an institutional investigation (Figure 12.1, www.publicationethics.org; ICMJE, 2008).

Fabrication or falsification of data

The recent case of Dr. Scott Reuben, an anaesthesiologist and pain management specialist who fabricated data in more than 21 studies of post-operative knee replacement patients, resulted in the retraction of more than 20 articles in the journal *Anaesthesia & Analgesia*, payment of fines and restitution totalling more than $400,000 and a jail sentence of 6 months (Borrell, 2009; Marcus, 2010).

One of the 'red flags' noticed in hindsight included a study in 2008 where Dr. Reuben claimed to have enrolled 200 patients undergoing knee replacement surgery yet he operated in an institution where only 'a handful' of these procedures is performed each year (Marcus, 2010). In fact, it was revealed during the investigation that he had enrolled no patients in that study and the data were all fabricated.

Although this case appears unique, a recent study of retractions in the medical literature (Steen, 2011b) revealed that deliberate scientific misconduct is perpetrated by a few 'repeat offenders' and retractions clustered in a relatively small number of journals. Additionally, these repeat offenders are unlikely, voluntarily, to identify every fraudulent article they have written (Sox and Rennie, 2006). A meta-analysis of survey data on the extent of scientific misconduct, excluding plagiarism, revealed nearly 2% of researchers admitted to fabricating or falsifying data and another 34% admitted to engaging in other questionable research practices themselves, but claimed 14% of their colleagues falsified data and 74% engaged in questionable research practices (Fanelli, 2009). The implications of this dilemma are that once fraud, fabrication or falsification have been identified in the body of work of an author, all articles written by that author or group of authors should be treated as suspect

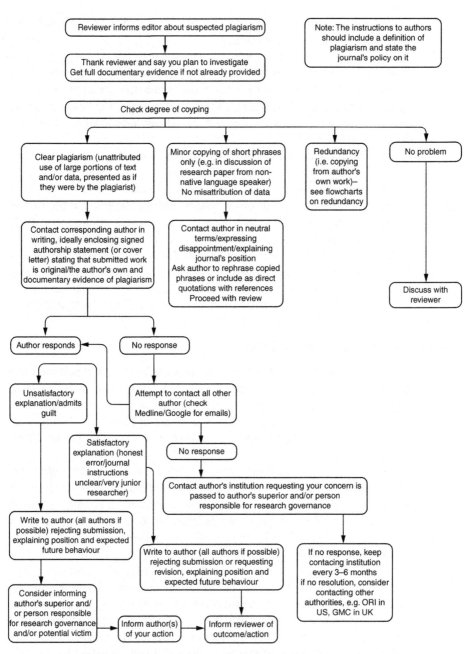

Figure 12.1 COPE flowchart for suspected plagiarism in a submitted manuscript. (© 2008 Committee on Publication Ethics. Used with permission (http://publicationethics.org/resources/flowcharts).)

until an investigation proves otherwise (Figure 12.1, www.publicationethics.org; Sox and Rennie, 2006).

Retracted articles present a continuing problem to researchers, a problem that continues to unfold as more meta-analyses and systematic reviews are conducted. Inclusion of duplicate studies or studies with fabricated data distorts the outcome of the meta-analysis. It is not always clear why an article is retracted based on the retraction notice (Wager and Williams, 2010). One of the largest groups involved in systematic reviews and meta-analyses is the Cochrane Library. Vlassov and Groves (2010) noted that five Cochrane Reviews in 2010 mentioned data fabrication, two mentioned data falsification and one mentioned plagiarism as reasons for excluding primary studies from reviews. In a move towards greater author accountability, some journals are requiring authors to confirm the extent of their involvement in the conduct of the research and the preparation of a manuscript (Rennie et al., 2000). The ICMJE (2008) specifically state that all authors must be able to defend the entire work publicly. These efforts are in service of forcing co-authors to be more accountable for data collection and analysis and catching some of the repeat offender first authors before the cases cause extensive 'ripples in the pond' (Wrobbel, 2007).

Case study 3   Fabricated data in a submitted manuscript

COPE case 01-08 (http://www.publicationethics.org/case/suspected-data-fabrication; Accessed 7 December 2011) illustrates the role of a reviewer in the discovery of possible data fabrication.

A manuscript was received from a group of authors who had published in a variety of other journals but not submitted to the journal in question before. The reviewer recommended rejection and in a covering letter to the editor stated that not only was the experimental design flawed, but he was also convinced that the experiment described had never been done. He had scanned Medline 1997–2001 and found seven other similar papers with a similar protocol, but in each case the authors had used a different substance. Each study included 40 subjects who were given either a supplement or control substance over a period of 1 year, which calculated to over 300 subjects recruited for these studies, and the possibility that several studies were conducted at the same time. The reviewer concluded that this was nearly impossible to achieve given the rigid entry criteria for the study, the rigorous protocol and potential difficulty in obtaining informed consent.

Although the paper was rejected and not published, the journal editor did attempt to contact the authors and the institution without success. The reviewer should be commended for the extra effort to follow up on his suspicions with a search of the literature for other studies by the same authors, although he should be protected by anonymity in any correspondence with the authors or the institution unless he consents otherwise. A difficulty for journal editors is that they have no recourse when a manuscript is rejected and to contact other journal editors who had previously published work by this group could be construed as slander because there is no evidence that this was not the first case of data fabrication. This differs from the Reuben case mentioned previously where ten suspect manuscripts had been published in one journal (Borrell, 2009).

Image manipulation

Manipulation of figures to create a false impression of data is a special case of data fabrication and cause for retractions in scientific publications. The Council of Science Editors (Scott-Lichter et al., 2009) has published guidelines for detecting image manipulation, which basically rely on direct examination of image files. This examination requires familiarity with programs such as Adobe Photoshop® to determine if selected features of the image have been differentially enhanced or obscured with the result that a false picture is created. The ORI (http://ori.hhs.gov/tools/; Accessed 7 December 2011) provides several forensic tools for use in image scanning that can be helpful for detecting image manipulation. Images that have been previously published cannot be used without permission of the copyright holder and appropriate acknowledgement. Authors must be prepared to provide original data if requested by an editor.

Finding retracted papers

Identifying which papers have been retracted from the literature and why is not an easy task. The retraction is permanently linked to the original article in the Medline database, and the original article remains accessible.

Activity 1

To access a list of retracted articles go to http://www.ncbi.nlm.nih.gov/pubmed and find the column labelled 'PubMed Tools'. Select 'Topic-Specific Queries' and scroll down to 'Additional Search Queries/Interfaces' and select 'Retracted Publication'. A list of all retracted publications (currently over 1900) appears that can be sorted by the following parameters: recently added, publication date, first author, last author, journal and title.

Inserting the term nursing in the search box identified 24 articles that had been retracted from various journals between 1993 and 2010, including those of one author identified by the ORI in the United States (http://www.ncbi.nlm.nih.gov/pubmed?term=retracted%20publication%20% 5Bpt%5D%20nursing; Accessed 5 December 2012).

Therefore, it is possible to find the retracted articles by Reuben by sorting alphabetically and guessing on which page the author's name will be found. There is also a link on the citation page to articles that have cited the retracted article. It is, however, quite common that retracted articles are cited even after retraction and the fault may be with the system (Sox and Rennie, 2006), possibly because not all articles are located through the PubMed search engine.

Publishers' databases or other search engines may not link retraction statements to the retracted articles; a circulating paper copy of the article will not give any indication that the article has been retracted. Checking every article in a systematic review against the PubMed list of retracted articles is time consuming yet the ICMJE (2008), section IV.A.9 states 'Authors are responsible for checking that none of the references cite retracted articles except in the context of referring to the retraction' (p. 13). The simplest way to accomplish this task is to enter every article title into the PubMed search field and find the official record of publication. Any retractions, errata, corrigenda or statements of concern (see Box 12.1) will be permanently linked to the publication record.

The ORI in the United States of America reports publicly on individuals who have been found guilty of research misconduct (see http://ori.hhs.gov/; Accessed 5 December 2011). The COPE website also has guidance on the retraction of articles by editors and publishers (see guidance paper at http:/ /publicationethics.org/files/u661/Retractions_COPE_gline_final_3_Sept_09_ 2_.pdf; Accessed 5 December 2011).

Box 12.1 Definitions of types of corrections to published articles

An *erratum* is a correction of an error not sufficient to cause any change in the interpretation of the work (e.g. table headings or misspellings).

A *corrigendum* is a correction of errors of greater significance that might cause a reinterpretation of the work (e.g. re-analysis of data reflecting changes to part of the findings and interpretation).

A *statement of concern* is a notice made by the publisher that there may be a problem with the work and an investigation is forthcoming (e.g. allegations of data fabrication have been received but findings from investigation are pending).

A *retraction* is a statement by the publisher that 'removes' the work from the scientific record for serious problems such as research or publishing misconduct (e.g. a duplicate article is retracted while the original or first published article remains intact).

Plagiarism

Plagiarism occurs when authors present the work of someone else as their own and without proper acknowledgement. The work of others could include words/text, data, theories, pictures, music or other media. To qualify as plagiarism, the content does not have to be copyrighted or trademarked; for example a faculty member who appropriates a student's idea and creates a manuscript from the student's work is guilty of plagiarism. This example of plagiarism is very difficult to prove and would likely go unrecognised except by the student. The more common scenario is illustrated by the case that follows.

> ### Case study 4   Plagiarism in a submitted manuscript
>
> A sole author, Dr. N, submitted a manuscript to a nursing journal that appeared to be a capstone project for an academic degree. The cover letter stated that the work was original and submitted in accordance with the guidelines for authors and conformed to the ICMJE authorship criteria. The journal routinely submits all submissions to a commercial plagiarism detection service, iThenticate®, which screens text for similarity with other published work. The similarity index on this submission exceeded 50% even when small matches and bibliography were excluded. Large blocks of verbatim text taken from six published articles constituted the majority of verbatim overlap.

Not all journals submit all articles to plagiarism detection software, but it is increasingly becoming the norm. By screening manuscripts on submission, reviewers are spared from wasting time on a manuscript that cannot be published even if favourably reviewed. The journal submission process should clearly state how manuscripts are processed and what will happen if unacceptable overlap occurs.

The COPE flowchart (http://www.publicationethics.org/resources/flow charts) titled *Suspected plagiarism in a submitted manuscript* gives detailed guidance for editors on how to handle this situation. In the case described, the author was notified by the managing editor and asked for an explanation but he/she never replied. The COPE flowchart (see Figure 12.1 – What to do if you suspect plagiarism in a submitted manuscript) suggests that the editor should go further and notify the author's institution or supervisor, but in reality, editors do not have time or staff to follow through on such an action. When follow up does occur, evidence of serious sanctions has appeared in publishing and academic circles, including retraction of published articles and retraction of Doctoral degrees by some universities (http://retractionwatch.wordpress.com).

Self-plagiarism easily occurs in some situations and is generally not acceptable. For example researchers who use a particular theoretical model or methodology may have difficulty finding new ways to write those sections in multiple manuscripts; therefore, a certain amount of overlap is expected. Self-plagiarism can rise to the level of redundant or duplicate publication if, in addition to verbatim overlap, the manuscript reuses previously published data even if the attempt is to reach a new audience as illustrated in the next case.

Many publishers have now signed up to use a common commercial plagiarism detection tool across all their journals. This tool is called CrossCheck/iThenticate: http://www.ithenticate.com/ (Accessed 5 December 2011). This link informs you who the current members of this product are and you can see the names of some of the major publishing agencies who have joined together in this common cause to ensure confidence in the scientific research community.

Case study 5   Duplicate publication

The author, Dr. X, had submitted a manuscript with significant overlap to a journal where she had published previously. Because the overlap was so significant (85%), in addition to rejecting the manuscript without further review, the editor researched the author's previous submission from several years earlier and found a very similar article in a journal from an entirely unrelated field. Comparison of the published articles revealed approximately 75% of the two articles were identical, but more importantly, the articles reported exactly the same data without any additional analyses.

The author in this case was notified in accordance with the COPE flowchart 'What to do if you suspect redundant (duplicate) publication in a published article'. The articles were retracted and because federally funded research was involved, the case was investigated by the author's university.

The implications of duplicate publication of research results have been discussed previously, but research universities that accept government money are also obligated to investigate these allegations and misconduct may be sanctioned by the ORI. These sanctions can include fines, termination, banishment from future funding and even jail.

Accidental or involuntary plagiarism is recognised in the COPE flowcharts as something that can occur when authors are not native speakers of the language in which they are writing. To be considered accidental or involuntary, the amount of copying should be relatively minor, but it should be resolved by the authors with editing or writing assistance from a native language speaker. Paraphrasing seems to be a skill that many students have never learned and may contribute to plagiarism. For authors with limited English language writing skills, the *Paraphrase: Write it in Your Own Words* module of the Purdue Online Writing Lab (http://owl.english.purdue.edu/owl/resource/619/01/) is a useful resource.

Summary and conclusions

Publication misconduct is a serious issue that can result in severe sanctions with the potential to ruin a reputation and a career. The process of writing to achieve educational and career goals can be fraught with frustration and disappointment, and novice authors may not receive the mentoring they need to navigate the process smoothly. Reviewers provide critical input to the editorial process by reporting suspected plagiarism of ideas and misrepresentation of current theory and practice.

Whether the reviewers are 'blinded' peer reviewers from a journal (see Chapter 11) or personally selected by the author for a pre-publication review, providing an honest and thoughtful critique is a professional responsibility. Plagiarism detection software can help authors and editors avoid intentional or accidental plagiarism. Authors who are confronted with unwarranted requests for guest authorship should respond that ethically, journal guidelines do not permit such actions. Nurses who are approached to be authors of sponsored articles should insist on full participation in the development of the article, legitimately, to claim authorship according to ethical guidelines. Nurse authors who apply ethical problem-solving behaviours to questions of authorship, reviewing and the conduct of research will avoid the possibility of sanctions and help protect the integrity of the scholarly record.

References

Borrell, B. (2009) A medical madoff: anesthesiologist faked data in 21 studies. Scientific American. Available at: http://www.scientificamerican.com/article.cfm?id=a-medical-madoff-anesthestesiologist-faked-data [Accessed 23 April 2012].

Fanelli, D. (2009) How many scientists fabricate and falsify research? A systematic review and meta-analysis of survey data. *PLoS ONE*, 4(5), e5738. doi:10.1371/journal.pone.0005738.

Godlee, F. (2011) Institutional and editorial misconduct in the MMR scare. *BMJ*, 342: d378. doi: 10.1136/bmj.d378.

Lo, B. & Field, M.J. (2009) Conflict of Interest in Medical Research, Education, and Practice. Committee on Conflict of Interest in Medical Research, Education, and Practice, Board on Health Sciences Policy Institute of Medicine of the National Academies. Washington, DC: National Academies Press.

Marcus, A. (2010) Reuben sentenced in fraud case. *Anesthesiology News*, 36(6). Available at: http://www.anesthesiologynews.com/ViewArticle.aspx?d=Web%2BExclusives&d_id=175&i=June%2B2010&i_id=637&a_id=15399&ses=ogst [Accessed 23 April 2012].

O'Neil, E.H. (2011) Through a glass darkly: reflections on change in health care, nursing, and blue ribbon committees. *Journal of Nursing Education*, 49(6), 318–321.

Office of Research Integrity (ORI) (2000) Managing allegations of scientific misconduct: A guidance document for editors. Office of Research Integrity, Office of Public Health and Science, U.S. Department of Health and Human Services. Available at: http://ori.hhs.gov [Accessed 23 April 2012].

Rennie, D., Flanagin, A. & Yank, V. (2000) The contributions of authors. *Journal of the American Medical Association*, 284(1), 89–91.

Scott-Lichter, D. & Editorial Policy Committee, Council of Science Editors. (2009) CSE's White Paper on Promoting Integrity in Scientific Journal Publications, 2009 Update. Reston, VA.

Sieber, J. (2006) Quality and value: how can we research peer review? *Nature*, doi: 10.1038/nature05006. Available at: http://www.nature.com/nature/peerreview/debate/op2.html[Accessed 28 April 2011].

Sox, H. & Rennie, D. (2006) Research misconduct, retraction, and cleansing the medical literature: lessons from the Poehlman case. *Annals of Internal Medicine*, 144(8), 609–613.

Steen, G. (2011a) Retractions in the medical literature: how many patients are put at risk by flawed research? *The Journal of Medical Ethics*, 37, 688–692.

Steen, G. (2011b) Retractions in the medical literature: who is responsible for scientific integrity? *American Medical Writers Association Journal*, 26(1), 2–7.

The PLoS Medicine Editors (2009) A new year's wish list for authors, reviewers, readers – and ourselves. *PLoS Medicine*, 6(12), e1000203. doi: 10.1371/journal.pmed.1000203.

US Senate Committee on Finance Sen. Grassley, C.E. (2010) *Ghostwriting in Medical Literature*. Minority Staff Report, 111th Congress, United States Senate.

Vlassov, V. & Groves, T. (2010) The role of Cochrane Review authors in exposing research misconduct (Editorial). *The Cochrane Library*. Available at: http://www.thecochranelibrary.com/details/editorial/886689/The-role-of-Cochrane-Review-authors-in-exposing-research-and-publication-miscond.html [Accessed 8 June 2012].

Wager, E. & Williams, P. (2010) Why and how do journals retract articles? An analysis of medline retractions 1988–2008. *Journal of Medical Ethics*, doi: 10.1136/jme.2010.040964. Available at: http://jme.bmj.com/content/early/2011/04/12/jme.2010.040964.short?q=w_jme_ah [Accessed 30 April 2011].

Wrobbel, E.D. (2007) Ripples in the pond: the wide-spread effects of a plagiarism disaster. *Plagiary: Cross-Disciplinary Studies in Plagiarism, Fabrication, and Falsification*, 52–56.

Websites

Retraction Watch "Tracking retractions as a window into the scientific process" is a blog launched August 2010. Available at: http://retractionwatch.wordpress.com/ [Accessed 23 April 2012].

The UK Research Integrity Office is an independent advisory body, providing guidance and support on good research practice and how to address fraud and misconduct in research. Launched in 2006, we provide assistance to researchers, research organisations and members of the public. Available at: http://www.ukrio.org/home [Accessed 23 April 2012].

The Office of Research Integrity (ORI) oversees and directs Public Health Service (PHS) research integrity activities on behalf of the Secretary of Health and Human Services with the exception of the regulatory research integrity activities of the Food and Drug Administration. Available at: http://ori.hhs.gov [Accessed 23 April 2012].

The International Committee of Medical Journal Editors (ICMJE) was formed in 1978 to develop uniform requirements for bio-medical journals. Available at: http://www.icmje.org [Accessed 23 April 2012]. Uniform Requirements for Manuscripts Submitted to Biomedical Journals: Writing and Editing for Biomedical Publication (Updated October 2008). Publication Ethics: Sponsorship, Authorship and Accountability International Committee of Medical Journal Editors.

The World Association of Medical Editors was established in 1995 as a voluntary association of editors of peer-reviewed medical journals. Available at: http://www.wame.org/about [Accessed 23 April 2012].

The Committee on Publication Ethics (COPE) was established in 1997 and is open to editors, publishers and others interested in publication ethics. Available at: http://publicationethics.org [Accessed 23 April 2012].

The International Academy of Nursing Editors (INANE) was established in 1982 to promote best practices in publishing and high standards in the nursing literature. Available at: http://www.nursingeditors-inane.org/index.html [Accessed 23 April 2012].

Nurse Author & Editor is a quarterly publication for nurse authors, editors and reviewers, first published in 1991. Registration is required but there is no fee. Available at: http://www.nurseauthoreditor.com/default.asp? [Accessed 23 April 2012].

Chapter 13
The World Wide Web and Its Potential for Publication

Paul Murphy and Seamus Cowman

Royal College of Surgeons in Ireland, Dublin, Ireland

Introduction to web publishing

Over the past decade, there has been a revolution in scholarly communication and publishing with a global shift to electronic publication. The World Wide Web has had a profound effect on all forms of popular and scholarly publication and we are currently in the midst of a continuing global transformation in all forms of communication. A multiplicity of web-based platforms and novel communication channels now enable individuals to communicate on a global scale in personal, social and professional domains. While many journals continue to appear in both electronic and print formats, the web format is generally the primary publication, especially in science, technology and medicine. Researchers and practitioners have welcomed easy global access to unprecedented numbers of journals in all disciplines. Web publishing has created new patterns of intensive use of electronic journals accessed through a variety of routes (Research Information Network, 2011). In terms of web publication, three areas of activity may be seen:

(1) Scholarly and research publications in science, technology and medicine have shifted almost completely to electronic publication.
(2) 'Grey literature' publications produced by non-commercial agencies, such as governments, public bodies, academic and professional groups, are now migrating rapidly from print.
(3) It is an emerging area of peer-to-peer and practitioner publication, both formal and informal, communicated through web channels such as blogs, social media and self-publishing sites.

The advantages of electronic publication are now well established. Users benefit from wide dissemination, ease of access '24/7', speed of publication

Writing for Publication in Nursing and Healthcare: Getting It Right, First Edition.
Edited by Karen Holland and Roger Watson.

and easy search and discovery through search engines and portal sites. A decade ago, nursing professionals were predicting that a major impact of electronic publishing would be to foster a new collaboration between readers and authors as comments, notes, corrections or rebuttals could be regularly added to articles, enhancing the long-term value of a work (Ludwick and Glazer, 2000). Unlike static print publications, electronic journals can be interactive and can be enhanced over time. The idea of a 'threaded' electronic publication with additional data, impossible to provide for in print, was proposed in 1999 (Chalmers and Altman, 1999). Additional added value predicted at the time included pre-publication of articles, multimedia content, additional data and supplements and embedded links and citations; many of these are now established features of electronic journals.

These benefits have driven the migration from print to electronic and have led to exponential growth in the use of e-journals and databases over two decades. New journal titles, both specialist and multi-disciplinary, continue to emerge. In addition to new content, reader behaviour has also adapted to the new electronic environment as key words through search engines, gateways and general bibliographic databases searching overtakes browsing via access though publisher sites (Tenopir, 2003; Williams et al., 2010).

Publications of international agencies, governments, charitable institutions, special interest groups and professional bodies are now often freely available on the Internet. Also available are material such as report and statistical series, conference and seminar proceedings, technical documentation and official papers of all kinds, often called the 'grey literature' (Alberani et al., 1990). In particular, the web offers enormous potential for lower costs in the production and dissemination of grey literature than the cumbersome and expensive production of hard copy reports. As a medium, the web has driven change in scholarly and practitioner communication globally.

Whether static print or electronic, academic research work is distinguished by the editorial and peer-review processes designed to assure publication of work of the highest calibre and quality. Traditional publications have retained all the quality assurance and peer-review processes while migrating to the web. New journals, which were born digitally, have also adopted traditional peer-review processes where appropriate. What is significant is that web publishing has generally speeded up the time cycle considerably. The past decade has seen both small and large publishers launch many new journals and publishers have developed new access models. Open access publishing has been the most significant development in the web era and has arisen in response to issues within the traditional publishing model and the economics of the publishing industry.

In the traditional model, authors and researchers freely contribute to journal content and to the peer-review process. On acceptance of an author's work for publication, the author generally relinquishes copyright of the work to the journal publisher. The publisher reformats the work for publication and sells the work back to readers who are required to pay a subscription fee to read it. Critics of this model argue that the research community freely contributes in authoring content and therefore that work should be freely available.

> ### Activity 1
>
> Check out the following publisher websites for information regarding article copyright and how authors are actually able to use their published work (traditional model of publication). You will see that there are variations in this area, certainly from use of the author's own work in scholarly endeavours:
> - *Elsevier*: http://www.elsevier.com/wps/find/authorsview.authors/rights
> - *Sage*: http://www.sagepub.com/authors/journal/permissions.sp
> - *Slack Corporation*: http://www.slackinc.com/permissions/faq.asp#2
> - *Wiley-Blackwell*: http://authorservices.wiley.com/bauthor/faqs_copyright.asp

Both commercial and scholarly publishers argue that they incur considerable costs in journal production and dissemination and that the subscription model is therefore necessary. Decades of high journal pricing has created significant barriers to access, as many journals are unaffordable to individuals or to institutions. Open access proposes a potential solution from the perspective of the users as it guarantees that access is free at the point of use.

Open access publishing and open access self-archiving

Scholarly research is a collaborative process and openness and exchange is the basis of knowledge advancement. One of the primary principles of open access is that wide dissemination of scholarly output is desirable from a number of dimensions. One aspect is that free, un-priced access at the point of use aids dissemination of knowledge from researcher to practitioner (Chan et al., 2009a). A related principle is a public benefit argument. The public and professional communities should have open access to research that is fully or partially funded by public funds. Finally, providing global open access promotes equity and development by enabling poorer institutions or poorer nations to retrieve information, which would otherwise be unaffordable due to the high costs charged by publishers (Chan et al., 2009b).

Authors have several options in terms of web publishing and open access (Table 13.1):

- Submission of work (articles, conference papers) for traditional publication in a subscription journal, where the publisher controls all access.
- 'Green' route open access, where an author submits a work for publication but also makes a pre-print or post-print copy of the work available in an open access archive, known as 'self-archiving'.

Table 13.1 Author's publishing options for a journal article.

	Green route open access		Gold route open access	Non-open access
Author	Manuscript preparation and potential journal selection		Manuscript preparation and potential journal selection	Manuscript preparation and potential journal selection
Author	Manuscript submission (pre-print copy)	Load pre-print copy to Institutional repository	Manuscript submission (pre-print copy)	Manuscript submission (pre-print copy)
Publisher	Peer review, correction and acceptance		Peer review, correction and acceptance	Peer review, correction and acceptance
Author	(Post-print copy)	*or* load post-print copy to institutional repository	(Post-print copy)	(Post-print copy)
Publisher	Published in journal		Published in journal	Published in journal
Reader	Subscriber access only	Open access to all	Open access to all	Subscriber access only

- 'Gold' route open access, where an author or an institution pays a fee to the publisher at time of publication and readers are free to view the work without any fee payable.

'Pre-prints' are manuscript copies of the work prior to peer-review or publisher correction. 'Post-prints' are the final copies post review and copy corrected for publication. Self-archiving of pre-prints makes work openly available in parallel to a published version, but self-archiving is not in itself publishing. Web repositories may be institutionally based in a university or research body or they may be geographically or subject-based collections.

Journals publishing open access work are distinguished by two levels of access:

(1) Full open access publishing, where an entire journal with all articles are available free to all on the web.
(2) Hybrid open access publication, whereby a journal publishes some articles that are freely available, while other articles in the same journal are priced.

Authors may consider that long-term open access to their published research will be a significant factor in selecting a journal. There may be institutional or funder imperatives that support a choice for long-term open access to the published work. In an academic climate of 'publish or perish', there may also be self-interest considerations based upon a greater visibility or impact of works publicly available.

The SOAP (Study of Open Access Publishing) project recently surveyed the range of offerings to authors by publishers and reported a continuing increase in open access publishing, especially in science, technology and medicine (Dallmeier-Tiessen et al., 2010; Vogel, 2011). It is argued that open access publishing combined with self-archiving optimises discoverability and accessibility of research articles by offering authors the possibility of greater use and higher impact until the ultimate goal of 100% free open access is finally achieved (Harnad et al., 2008).

Activity 2

Find out what your organisation has access to in terms of open access journals. If you work in a university, obtain a copy of the guidance for submission of your research outputs and funded project reports into the Repository (see Section 'Depositing in a repository'). Find out by searching one of the major web portals like Google, how many of the outputs in the repository you are able to access. It is also possible in Google Scholar, for example, to also determine how many times that work has been cited by others.

BioMed Central

BioMed Central (http://www.biomedcentral.com) is an open access publisher that operates entirely online and all journals and papers are freely available.

Activity 3

Access this website and familiarise yourself with the guidance pages for authors.

Online submission and electronic review leads to an efficient and speedy production process. For nursing authors it does open up new and different opportunities for publication and given the high visibility and open access, it is likely that your paper will be accessed by large numbers of people. Because it is an exclusively online publication there is unlimited space for tables, photos and video footage.

A major difference between BioMed Central and other form of journal publication is that the author retains copyright of the paper through the paper being licensed under a creative commons license. A creative commons licence (http://creativecommons.org/licenses/; Accessed 30 November 2011) enables appropriate reuse of copyright work by authors and by readers. It could be placed on your personal or institutional home page, could be translated and distributed to others in any form; you have the opportunity to promote your paper through many avenues – email lists, online links and conferences. Many of the BioMed Central 207 open access journals have been accepted by Thomson Reuters for citation tracking and inclusion on the Web of Science.

Regular email alerts and updates are provided to over 500,000 registered users. One BioMedNet Central title, *BMC Nursing*, is one of the most widely known open access journals in nursing and has been in production since 2002. *BMC Nursing* publishes research articles after full peer review and is indexed by PubMed, CAS, EMBASE, Scopus, CINAHL and Google Scholar.

Publishers with nursing journals have been slow to enter electronic publishing and even slower to adopt open access. Publishers continue to offer high-quality titles from the print era but there are also some new journal titles emerging. UlrichsWeb (http://www.ulrichsweb.com/ulrichsweb), a global serials directory, records 480 currently publishing journals in the subject category 'nursing', of which 228 are refereed titles. There 29 nursing journals classified as 'open access', 15 of which are refereed. In the online directory of journals, DOAJ, the Directory of Open Access (and Hybrid) Journals (http://www.opendoar.org), there are 40 nursing journals listed as open access with a variety of free, author fee or hybrid models.

Publication fees

Open access web-published journals have publication costs like any other journal. Editorial, design, production, marketing and maintenance costs must all be met. Publishers add significant value within the current system in providing authors with quality assurance, editorial services, peer review, assured dissemination and archiving. Publication fees represent a new model in scholarly publishing where the production cost is shifted from the readers at the point of use to the authors at the point of production. Many open access journals charge publication fees or article processing fees payable on article acceptance; other open access journals, especially professional society journals, do not charge authors directly but have alternative funding models (Suber, 2008). Publishing fees vary widely between publishers, between disciplines and between different journals. In some cases, fees may be discounted or waived for authors from developing countries.

As an example, one of the most widely known open access journals in nursing is the BioMedNet Central title, *BMC Nursing*, and as of 2011, the publication fee per article published is US$1820/€1365, payable by the authors on acceptance of the article by the journal. This rate may be discounted significantly as there are various institutional membership and support options available for BMC, which may reduce the direct fee payable by the authors. An example of the costs involved to potential authors can be seen in Box 13.1. The BMC Nursing charges similar fees but slightly different guidance (see Box 13.2).

One example of an open access article in this journal, including access to a pdf version is: Higginbottom, G. (2011) The transitioning experiences of internationally educated nurses into a Canadian healthcare system: a focused ethnography, BMC, 10, 14. http://www.biomedcentral.com/content/pdf/1472-6955-10-14.pdf.

The *Journal of Nursing Management* is an example of a hybrid subscription journal where the publisher offers authors the option of paying a publication fee to ensure that a specific article is free to all readers. This is called Online Open (see http://olabout.wiley.com/WileyCDA/Section/id-406241.html).

As an author, it may be useful to consider at an early stage the publication fee factor in scoping potential journal titles for publication. If you are undertaking a research bid to major funding bodies it is important that funding for this option and the one such as BMC Medicine are factored into the bidding proposals. For BMC Medicine article processing charge see Box 13.1.

Peer review, quality, timeliness and impact

As a goal of open access is to deliver quality research content but without the barrier of affordability, maintaining quality assurance is a key success factor. Open access publishers generally deploy the same peer-review procedures as those used by subscription journals. Authors rate the quality of peer-review

Table 13.2 Main advantages and disadvantages to nursing authors – open access versus non-open access.

Open access		Non-open access	
Advantage	**Disadvantage**	**Advantage**	**Disadvantage**
Speed of publication	Limited range of journals published	Larger range of journals	Slower process to publication
Availability through the web	Lower impact factor	Established traditional system	Publisher may embargo free publication
No cost to the reader	Significant cost to the author	No cost to author	Possible subscriber access only
Retention of copyright		Higher impact factor	No copyright ownership
Open access to all with possible increased citation			

and publisher reputation as important factors in selecting a journal for article submission. Another established advantage of open access is that the time-line from article acceptance to publication and availability is much shorter than with subscription journals (Harnad, 1996; Pappalardo et al., 2008) (see Table 13.2).

Research impact is a critical issue for researchers, universities, funders and publishers. While individuals aspire to publish in a journal with a good repu-tation and a high impact factor as noted, for example by Thomson Reuter's ISI (see http://thomsonreuters.com/products_services/science/free/essays/impact_factor/), on a larger scale the value of research outputs is being for-mally assessed and compared in countries worldwide, for example Australia (http://www.arc.gov.au/era/era_2012/era_2012.htm; Accessed 16 December 2011).

Harnad et al. (2008) state that an article's research impact is:

[T]he degree to which its findings are read, used, applied, built upon and cited by researchers in their own further research and applications. Research impact is a measure of the progress and the productivity of research.
(Harnad et al., 2008, p. 36)

It is further claimed that impact relates not only to the quality of the work but to whether the article is readily accessible and if it is, therefore, more likely to be cited in the future.

Measurement of the research impact of electronic publications in either open access journals or institutional repositories can be problematic. Early studies appear to show a correlation between open access status and subsequent increased citation counts (Harnad et al., 2008; Pappalardo et al., 2008).

This raises questions of an open access advantage through increased citation rates; or are there other factors involved, such as rapid availability of self-archived items or of authors selecting higher quality work for open access archiving? Some studies have reported that citation rates for refereed post-prints are in many instances higher than subscription only publication in certain disciplines (Gargouri et al., 2010).

Others have concluded that there is as yet no evidence for open access citation benefits considering the complexities of citation analysis and the considerable variations in metrics between different scholarly disciplines (Craig et al., 2007). Open access may reach more readers but the presumed citation advantage is not evident over time (Davis et al., 2008; Davis, 2010).

Many of the reported studies of research impact are in scientific and biomedical disciplines and currently there are no bibliometric studies of the nursing literature to indicate any impacts. The evidence for nursing simply does not exist yet, but as the increased browsing and reading of open access articles is an established trend in many disciples, the likelihood of an increased readership may be a factor the nursing author should consider in assessing the open access options.

Depositing in a repository

Repositories were created to enable authors to deposit and disseminate work as freely as possible and to enable users to access the content without any barriers. The Scholarly Publication and Academic Resources Coalition proposed that, while:

> [I]nstitutional repositories centralise, preserve, and make accessible an institution's intellectual capital, at the same time they will form part of a global system of distributed, interoperable repositories that provides the foundation for a new disaggregated model of scholarly publishing.
>
> (SPARC, 2002, p. 6)

Repositories are typically institutional services, especially in universities, but they may also be subject or country based. Repositories are growing rapidly worldwide with The Directory of Open Access Repositories (DOAR) showing growth to over 2000 services globally at end of 2010 (see http://www .opendoar.org/; Accessed 23 April 2012).

From the author's perspective, repositories have raised new issues about their work. An article may exist in three versions:

(1) Pre-print (pre-refereeing)
(2) Post-print (final draft post-refereeing)
(3) Publisher final (published copy)

This raises several important questions for authors to consider when preparing an article for publication, as it is no longer simply that the author guidelines are important to consider but also the issue of whether to publish in an open access journal, which may or may not require an 'upfront' financial payment of some kind or one where no subscription is required but access to the article is only possible if the end user or reader has access to the journal via either institutional or personal subscription.

For a member of staff in a university or a postgraduate research student in a university this becomes less of a problem, but there are potential authors without this access who are prepared to pay for their work to be published and accessible through the much more worldwide portal such as a Google or Google Scholar.

Some of the questions are: Does the publisher allow deposit of a copy in a repository and, if so, which version? What terms and use conditions will govern an author's work in a repository? Will the author's interests be protected and will the integrity of the work be safeguarded? While open access repositories do not perform peer review, they can contain peer-reviewed post-prints as easily as un-refereed pre-prints. An author can deposit a pre-print at the time a manuscript is submitted and can then deposit the post-print after it is published (Suber, 2006).

The benefits of maintaining an archive of self-deposited work in a secured repository ensures that an author can maintain and promote access to a complete body of work over time. In addition to copies indexed in journals by databases such as CINAHL and MEDLINE, open access copies will be fully discoverable by current and by future web search engines.

Currently, repository copies of works can be readily discovered works by author or institution name, for instance, or by subject key words via Google Scholar. Unlike many personal or corporate websites, repositories provide a structured environment for the content and are specifically designed to provide long-term security and preservation of an author's work. A distinct advantage of repositories is that they provide complete viewing and download data for authors, so that the readership and usage information is always known.

Your academic or service institution may have its own repository or may be collaborating in a network with other institutions. There may also be a policy or indeed a mandate in place in some institutions advising on self-archiving options or requirements. Institutional repository services, often managed by library services, generally offer full service support and advice to authors seeking to deposit their work. Such support will enable authors, speedily, to resolve seemingly complex copyright, licensing and use issues.

Standard tools such as open access licences like creative commons are widely in place to protect the rights of all parties, authors and users, in the appropriate use of self-archived material (see http://creativecommons .org/about; Accessed 23 April 2012). Repository managers are skilled in facilitating authors to make speedy choices from various options that may be available. Initially the whole process of self-archiving seemed bothersome and time consuming for some authors but repository deposit procedures continue to improve (Suber, 2006). The impact on nursing is difficult to judge as yet but a subject search of The DOAR (http://www.opendoar.org) retrieved over 720 documents under the term 'nursing'. On further examination, however, it is evident that many journals classed as nursing by some open access publishers publish little actual 'nursing' research.

Funding bodies and open access mandates

Under subscription publishing models, research outputs are privatised to publishers and articles have to be purchased by all subsequent users, individually or via their institutions. Research funders recognised open access as an opportunity to increase the effectiveness of the research by improving dissemination and maintaining communication between health researcher and practitioner (Chan et al., 2009a). This is particularly the case in the realm of publicly funded research where there is a need to ensure the advancement of research and development in the interests of society and health services for instance, without unnecessary duplication of research effort.

Much nursing research derives directly from funding bodies that are publicly funded or funded on a charitable basis. Funding bodies have an interest in encouraging funded researchers to provide public open access to their research outputs for a variety of reasons:

- All work becomes open and accessible.
- The funding body itself will have permanent access to funded work.
- There is a record of achievement reducing the risk of duplication.
- A clearer public benefit accrues from the investment in the research.

Across the globe, funding bodies are requiring that supported researchers publish results in open access journals or to self-archive in open repositories. Examples of major funding bodies with open access policies include the National Institutes of Health (US), the European Research Council, The Wellcome Trust (UK), Canadian Institutes of Health Research, and the Australian Research Council. Initially, funder policies tended to simply encourage authors to adopt open access solutions but voluntary systems are increasingly being replaced by mandatory compliance requirements (Pappalardo et al., 2008, Section 6.2). Where self-archiving in a repository may not be an option, some funders allow the use of support funds to pay author publication fees.

For grant-aided research, authors may need to establish the specific publishing policy of a funding body and what impact such policies may have on the choice of a journal for final publication. There may be conflicts arising between a funding body's open access mandate and a publisher's copyright terms and conditions, which might limit access or self-archiving options. In general terms, the funder's grant conditions apply to authors before they negotiate the publication stage. The author must ensure in advance that publisher copyright conditions are compatible with funder requirements (Pappalardo et al., 2008, Section 6.4). SHERPA RoMEO (http://www.sherpa.ac.uk/romeo/) is an invaluable service based at the university of Nottingham, UK, which enables an author to check funder and publisher compatibility and to discover what options individual journals permit in terms of self-archiving relative to funder mandates.

Electronic theses and dissertations

Master's theses and doctoral dissertations produced for university awards are a unique and valuable source of nursing research. When produced in print with single copies deposited in university libraries, theses are difficult to identify and even more difficult to access, effectively rendering an enormous body of work virtually useless. Authors rarely received recognition for valuable work as theses and dissertations were not read and not cited in the nursing literature.

Recently, there is a growing trend worldwide for university theses and dissertations to be submitted electronically. Electronic documents significantly increase the options available to authors by enabling a document to include sound, video and multimedia content. E-theses can link to other content and additional data can be easily attached to an electronic document. The university may then offer the graduate student options to make the full text of their work freely available immediately or to restrict access internally or for a specific period. The final theses, in portable document format, is archived in the institutional repository enabling the author to expose and share their thesis to a global readership.

We have seen that documents in repositories can be found using web portals and engines such as Google Scholar. Commercial publishers such as ProQuest have database products indexing theses, and the Networked Digital Library of Theses and Dissertations (NDLTD) is an organisation dedicated to supporting access to electronic theses. Goodfellow gives an overview of the benefits of electronic publication of theses for nurse scholars and calls for further development in open access for nursing research (Goodfellow, 2009). Macduff presents a useful case study evaluating the process and outcome in disseminating a nursing PhD dissertation (Macduff, 2009). Macduff encourages a proactive approach on the part of the nurse researcher to the e-thesis and presents evidence of the increased impact and readership electronic publication brings for the author.

Web publishing, patient information and best practice

The World Wide Web is a major source of health information for patients and for families. How engaged have nurses and healthcare professionals been in the development and delivery of Internet-based information? Nurses have been seen to have a significant role in interpreting and evaluating the multiplicity of web-published resources for patients and are challenged to incorporate web resources into patient support (Anderson and Klemm, 2008). It is less clear how active nurses have been in generating original patient support material. Healthcare advocacy and patient support agencies worldwide have established web publishing channels providing authoritative and reliable information for patients. Examples include the British Heart Foundation (www.bhf.org.uk) and the American Cancer Society (www.cancer.org).

Web publishing has been established in support of evidence-based practice. The US National Guideline Clearinghouse (www.guideline.gov) and NHS Evidence (www.evidence.nhs.uk) are both examples of web-based dissemination of best practice guidelines. On another more informal level, authors, readers and colleagues can flag and discuss practice issues in various peer-to-peer networks. Blogs and wikis for instance have been used in evidence-based and nurse education contexts. 'Blogs' refers to 'weblogs' and they are a flexible open source platform for collecting, presenting and publishing information.

Blogs typically operate like newsletters but ones where authors can create and publish web content with very little technical know how. Audiences may be a team of collaborators, colleagues in a hospital, a class of students or any public community of interest. Blogs may be focused quite narrowly as in the example of *Nursing Research: Show me the evidence!* (http://evidencebasednursing.blogspot.com). 'Wikis' are another web-based publishing platform designed to enable a collaborative work group to originate, edit and share documents. Wikis are useful for publication of the output of a specific collaboration and enable such work to be fully exposed to a web readership (Donovan and Bernardo, 2009).

Communities of interest

The web is also an informal channel wherein authors, readers and colleagues can flag and discuss new research in various peer-to-peer networks. The journal website is now but one place to access research articles. Web services such as wikis, podcasts, listservs, blogs and various other social media enable interest groups and online communities to quickly form and to share material. The new web services facilitate rapid peer-to-peer information exchange. The very informal nature of such information sharing makes it difficult to quantify and to measure the impact such activity.

Conclusion

In summary, there are advantages and disadvantages to both open access and non-open access publication (see Table 13.2). In addition, web publishing speeds up the entire publishing process. In the case of electronic journal articles, the period from manuscript deposit to copy revision to final acceptance may be measured in weeks. Time to actual publication and availability may also be a matter of weeks. Reader response and feedback may now occur immediately generating a more direct relationship between author and reader in the electronic environment. The shift from print journals and books to electronic versions has been a major transformative factor in scholarly communication over the past two decades. The future for publishing journals and books, as well as other forms of communication media will continue to challenge all of us to develop new skills in the dissemination of our research and innovations.

References

Alberani, V., De Castro Pietrangeli, P. & Mazza, A.M. (1990) The use of grey literature in health sciences: a preliminary survey. *Bulletin of the Medical Library Association*, 78(4), 358–363.

Anderson, A.S. & Klemm, P. (2008) The Internet: friend or foe when providing patient education? *Clinical Journal of Oncology Nursing*, 12(1), 55–63.

Chalmers, D. & Altman, D. (1999) How can medical journals help prevent poor medical research? Some opportunities presented by electronic publishing. *Lancet*, 353(9151), 490–493.

Chan, L., Arunachalam, S. & Kirsop, B. (2009a) The chain of communication in health science: from researcher to health worker through open access. *OpenMed*, 2009; 3(3), e111–e119. Available at: http://www.ncbi.nlm.nih.gov/pmc/articles/PMC2765774/ [Accessed 14 Jan 2011].

Chan, L., Arunachalam, S. & Kirsop, B. (2009b) Open access: a giant leap towards bridging health inequities. *Bulletin of the World Health Organization*, 87(8), doi: 10.1590/S0042-96862009000800021. Available at: http://www.scielosp.org/scielo.php?pid=S0042-96862009000800021&script=sci_arttext [Accessed 22 Jan 2011].

Craig, I., Plume, A., McVeigh, M., Pringle, J. & Amin, M. (2007) Do open access articles have greater citation impact? A critical review of the literature. *Journal of Informetrics*, v1(3), 239–248. doi: 10.1016/j.joi.2007.04.001.

Dallmeier-Tiessen, S., Darby, R., Goerner, B., Hyppoelae, J., Igo-Kemenes, P., Kahn, D., Lambert, S., Lengenfelder, A., Leonard, C., Mele, S., Polydoratou, P., Ross, D., Ruiz-Perez, S., Schimmer, R., Swaisland, M. & van der Stelt, W. (2010) First results of the SOAP project. Available at: http://arxiv.org/abs/1010.0506v1 [Accessed 22 December 2011].

Davis, P.M. (2010) Open access citations. Still robust after three years. *BMJ*, 341, c6854. doi: 10.1136/bmj.c6854.

Davis, P.M., Lewenstein, B.V., Simon, D.H., Booth, J.G. & Connolly, M.J. (2008) Open access publishing, article downloads, and citations: randomised controlled trial. *BMJ*, 337, a568. doi: 10.1136/bmj.a568.

Donovan, S. & Bernardo, L.M. (2009) The role of collaborative Web publishing tools in evidence-based practice. *Journal of Emergency Nursing*, 35(2), 149–150.

Gargouri, Y., Hajjem, C., Larivière, V., Gingras, Y., Carr, L., Brody, T. & Harnad, S. (2010) Self-selected or mandated, open access increases citation impact for higher quality research. *PLoS One*, 5(10), e13636. doi: 10.1371/journal.pone.0013636.

Goodfellow, L.M. (2009) Electronic theses and dissertations: a review of this valuable resource for nurse scholars worldwide. *International Nursing Review*, 56(2), 159–165.

Harnad, S. (1996) Implementing peer review on the Net: scientific quality control in scholarly electronic journals. In: Peek, R. & Newby, G. (Eds.), *Scholarly Publication: The Electronic Frontier.* Cambridge, MA: MIT Press, pp. 103-108. Available at: http://cogprints.org/1692/1/harnad96.peer.review.html [Accessed 12 December 2010].

Harnad, S., Brody, T., Vallièresc, F., Carr, L., Hitchcock, S., Gingras, Y., Oppenheim, C., Hajjem, C. & Hilfi, E.R. (2008) The access/impact problem and the green and gold roads to open access: an update. *Serials Review,* 34(1), 36-40. doi: 10.1016/j.serrev.2007.12.005.

Ludwick, R. & Glazer, G. (2000) Electronic publishing: the movement from print to digital publication. *Online Journal of Issues in Nursing,* 5(1), 2.

Macduff, C. (2009) An evaluation of the process and initial impact of disseminating a nursing e-thesis. *Journal of Advanced Nursing,* v65(5), 1010-1018.

Pappalardo, K.M., Fitzgerald, B.T., Fitzgerald, A.M., Kiel-Chisholm, S.D., Georgiades, J. & Austin, A.C. (2008) Understanding Open Access in the Academic Environment: A Guide for Authors (unpublished). Available at: http://eprints.qut .edu.au/14200/3/Understanding_Open_Access_in_an_Academic_Environment-_A_Guide_for_Authors_[web_version].pdf?bcsi_scan_9CF786ACA806128D=0& bcsi_scan_filename=Understanding_Open_Access_in_an_Academic_Environme nt_A_Guide_for_Authors_[web_version].pdf [Accessed 11 December 2010].

Research Information Network (2011) E-journals: their use, value and impact: final report. Research Information Network. Available at: http://www.rin.ac.uk/about [Accessed 23 April 2012].

SPARC (2002) The case for institutional repositories: A SPARC position paper. Available at: http://www.arl.org/sparc/bm~doc/ir_final_release_102.pdf [Accessed 15 January 2011].

Suber, P. (2006) Six things that researchers need to know about open access. SPARC Open Access Newsletter, Issue 94. Available at: http://www.earlham .edu/~peters/fos/newsletter/02-02-06.htm [Accessed 5 December 2010].

Suber, P. (2008) Open access in 2007. *Journal of Electronic Publishing,* 11(1), doi: 10.3998/3336451.0011.110.

Tenopir, C. (2003) Use and users of electronic library resources: an overview and analysis of recent research studies, Council on Library and Information Resources, Washington, DC. Available at: http://www.clir.org/pubs/reports/ pub120/pub120.pdf. [Accessed 5 December 2010].

Vogel, G. (2011) Open access gains support. *Fees and Journal Quality Deter Submissions Science,* 21 January 2011331(6015), 273. doi: 10.1126/science.331.6015.273-a.

Williams, P., Nicholas, D. & Rowlands, I. (2010) E-journal usage and impact in scholarly research: a review of the literature. *New Review of Academic Librarianship,* v16(2), 192-207. doi: 10.1080/13614533.2010.503645.

Further reading

De Groote, S. & Barrett, F. (2010) Impact of online journals on citation patterns of dentistry, nursing, and pharmacy faculty. *Journal of Medical Library Association,* 98(4), 305-308.

Eysenbach, G. (2006) Citation advantage of open access articles. *PLoS Biol,* 4(5), e157. doi: 10.1371/journal.pbio.0040157.

Chapter 14

Dissemination of Published Work: The Process and Value

Sue Turale

Yamaguchi University Graduate School of Medicine, Ube, Japan

Chapter aim

This chapter informs the reader of the value of, and some major issues involved in, disseminating results of project work, and sets out a variety of strategies for use in disseminating strategies to various audiences.

Introduction

Having read this far into the book, we hope that you will remain committed on your learning journey into the why, how, where and when of writing for publication. My goal in this chapter is to persuade you to think more deeply about the dissemination of the results of your project work and then take action to improve what you are currently doing to inform others about your results.

Unfortunately, healthcare professionals around the world, including nurses, often do not pay enough attention to getting their work distributed to the very audiences that need to know the outcome of their work. It could be because of the following:

- The project work has been completed but results have not been distributed at all.
- The results have been distributed but they have not reached the intended audience effectively.
- The results have been distributed to the intended audience, but have not been effectively translated into practice, either by health professionals or the consumers of healthcare.

Writing for Publication in Nursing and Healthcare: Getting It Right, First Edition.
Edited by Karen Holland and Roger Watson.
© 2012 John Wiley & Sons, Ltd. Published 2012 by John Wiley & Sons, Ltd.

Each of these scenarios is problematic and – ultimately – a waste of public or private money, and personal and professional investment by project team members. Simply put, they are detrimental to efforts to improve healthcare practices and the lives of the people whose health we are trying to help. When results of project work are not distributed effectively, this might also have a direct bearing on the quality and quantity of resources available to researchers in the future for their project work.

I use the term 'project work' in this chapter as a general term to include many types of scholarly work, including research, educational projects, clinical or management improvement activities and quality assurance work, since not all innovative results come from research projects. The main focus here, however, concerns the research that is meant to have an impact on healthcare. Too often, in many projects, there has been no early planning about *where* and *how* the end results should be distributed. This chapter is about getting you to think early in your planning processes about *why* it is important to disseminate your work, some of the *issues* involved in such dissemination and giving you some practical tips about distributing the results of your work. Let us focus firstly on the *why*, the value of dissemination.

The value of disseminating your work

By dissemination I mean communicating the innovative results of your project work to others. Dissemination can be either a systematic, highly planned process or it can be a passive, unplanned one. It can take many forms, either written or verbal. However, you should always remember that the passive, unplanned process is less likely to yield good results that make a difference to health outcomes and practices. Currently, there are more avenues of communication opening up as the world becomes cleverer at using technology (see Chapter 13), and there are growing efforts to improve the quality and safety of healthcare. But first you might ask: why bother to spread the results of your work?

Foremost, the value of dissemination of innovative knowledge is clearly related to the values we hold as health professionals. Nurses in practice are often reminded about their duty of care to their patients, and I am sure most of them like to think of themselves as ethical practitioners. The same is true for those of us who are working on various projects. As researchers, there should be no argument that we have a duty of care to science and health, and to the participants involved in our work. Disseminating knowledge to an audience is a vital part of research, and forms part of that duty of care. It is easy to understand that our participants, whether they are the general public, health professionals, institutions, patients, carers or families, might feel quite frustrated when they have engaged in our research but have not been informed of the results. Clearly, they have been interested enough to agree to join in our research, so our duty is to provide the results to them in an understandable and useful manner. If we do not, they will be less likely to be involved in future projects, and we are effectively excluding them from our new knowledge about health. Moreover, if we want to ensure that our findings are valid, then sharing results and getting feedback from participants should be part of the research process, both during and after a project.

Second, when thinking of the value of disseminating results, we need to think about the scarce resources that are available for project work in health services generally, and our accountability in using these. If you live in a developing country, project funding might be very scarce or even non-existent. In these times of global recession, even in relatively wealthy countries, project funds might still be scarce. If you have been in a competitive situation trying to get funding for your project, then you will know what I mean. As the effects of the worldwide recession go deeper, research funds shrink, so increasingly the guidelines of governments and non-government grants are becoming stricter. They want to make sure approved projects target health priorities and that these have tangible benefits for the health of the public and healthcare delivery. Therefore, in an ethical or moral sense, we have a duty of care to make sure that our project work is undertaken in a way that makes a difference to improving health, and, for example, has a focus on changing outdated clinical practice for the better.

Project grants are often from the public purse, so it is reasonable that researchers have a duty of care for these and are held accountable to the taxpayer for their use, including ensuring that they provide research results in a meaningful way to the intended audiences. With this in mind I hope you will agree that it is important that researchers take a planned approach to disseminating their results. It makes common sense that, if you can argue the merits of your project and how the results can be implemented, including providing results in a meaningful way to the audience you are targeting, then you will have more success in gaining funds. This then leads to the greater possibility that your research will have positive outcomes for health because you have clearly thought through the process of how you are going to distribute the findings. Moreover, good dissemination will help convince policy makers, the general public and health service providers to implement the findings of a project.

Another value in spreading the results of your findings is that these might help to foster other research-related activities (Cleary et al., 2007) by health professionals where there are gaps in knowledge and innovation. Often, research has to be replicated to confirm findings for various populations, but I do not mean that researchers need to keep researching the same things repeatedly, which is sometimes a problem in nursing. However, by using systematic review processes, the generalisability of research findings can be found and this leads to more confidence in implementing findings in practice that have solid research evidence from a variety of sources.

The process of disseminating the findings of your work and its outcomes

In getting you to think about how and where you are going to communicate the results of your work, I want to highlight some issues in dissemination.

These include timeliness of dissemination; problems in training researchers in dissemination methods; publishing only in journals; only presenting in conferences or workshops; reasons for the non-implementation and non-distribution of findings and the costs involved.

Publishing as dissemination of your work

Most of us realise that knowledge does not remain stagnant but, unfortunately, changes in healthcare practices are often slow because knowledge dissemination may be quite diffuse. As a journal editor I know that often 5–7 years can pass from the time that data are collected and analysed, and the findings published in a journal. It may take even longer if a book publication is involved. Many years can also pass before the information filters down into the healthcare setting and results are actually used to change practice; this is clearly disturbing. If we fail to spread important findings quickly, and these are not translated into practice appropriately and effectively, we are failing our patients by not improving timely access to modern healthcare techniques or knowledge. Changes in practice may be hindered because clinicians have not accessed nor implemented recent findings into their practice in a timely fashion. Part of the problem is that there has not been widespread research on effective strategies for disseminating information to the right audiences (Haines et al., 2004) and how that information can then be translated into practice.

Disseminating research results beyond academic and professional journals has often been a low priority among researchers (Cleary et al., 2007). Additionally, while researchers may be trained well in research methods and reporting their results in the literature, they often do not receive training about how to spread their results widely to the appropriate audience, a real problem in my view in education today. It is an indictment on our education systems that the research training has not emphasised the importance of teaching students practical ways of doing this, hence this chapter. Part of the problem lies in various curricula not reflecting research evidence, and educational activities being designed to ensure that all programs are connected to improving quality of care (Haines et al., 2004).

Today there is an increasing pressure on academics, graduate students and other researchers for publishing their work in high-impact journals. These are journals that have been deemed to be so by one source: The Thomson Reuter Journal Impact Factor, a product of Thomson ISI, which calculates, using quantitative measures, the citation data or number of times an article is cited by others in a given number of years. Each year they publish a list of the Impact Factor ratings for the journals that have been rated as of the standard to be in the citation database following a rigorous evaluation process (see http://thomsonreuters.com/products_services/science/free/essays/impact_factor/ for details of this product).

Competitive research grants often hinge on researchers having a history of high-impact publications, and academics in some countries today are often rewarded financially or through promotion for publishing in high-impact journals. Therefore, there may be very little incentive for such researchers to disseminate their findings more broadly because they have to be busy preparing for the next project in order to obtain funding, or there is no reward for publishing elsewhere.

If you are in a situation where you need to publish in a high-impact journal as a student or a health professional, do not be mistaken into thinking that achieving that goal is the end of your project work. You clearly need to think about how else you can inform others of your work in a way that is accessible, understandable and useful.

Another issue is that there is widespread evidence in both low- and high-income countries of a failure to implement health interventions that have been shown to be cost-effective through good research (Haines et al., 2004). Some of this non-implementation comes about because of: systematic failures within organisations to incorporate modern technical information; lack of resources in low-income countries; social and cultural issues, such as staff unwillingness to change practices or information not being culturally appropriate; or a lack of persuasion of decision-makers by health professionals to implement findings. In my experience, it is unusual for project granting bodies to fund the true cost of dissemination of project outcomes.

For example good dissemination strategies may involve attending conferences to present findings, facilitating and delivering workshops, producing pamphlets and information booklets, developing new guidelines and protocols for practice and so on. In some settings these are often costly strategies, and the time and resources have to be found somewhere if knowledge is to be spread and real implementation is to occur.

The written format of the dissemination information

The information that is released by the researchers may be in a form that is not understandable or acceptable to practitioners of healthcare. For example providing busy clinicians with a journal article that is heavily philosophical and theoretical, or interspersed with complex statistics and data analysis is not going to be understandable to most, and so will be disregarded. These clinicians may not have the training to understand the work and so lack the necessary critical appraisal skills. Busy work settings mean they do not have the time to try to digest the findings. They need and want to have results written in such a way that is understandable, and focused on the implications for their practice, hence the need for specific translational considerations. Clinicians often do not like to use research reports, may not access the Internet, and prefer to use and draw heavily on knowledge derived in the workplace, from patient care, colleagues and evidence-based protocols (Gerrish et al., 2011). Clearly, if you write up the results of your project in a journal or textbook that is not readily available or popular with your target audience, you will surely miss the opportunity to make a difference to practice. You need to think of better ways to inform them of your findings so they can use them in practice.

One way of doing this is to put your findings into a local or regional journal that has immediate cultural and social relevancy for the clinicians. Parker et al. (2010) in New South Wales, Australia cited many of the problems I have already mentioned about clinicians not accessing journal articles, or indeed writing them. This group of authors described the implementation of a local journal through co-operation between local health services and two local universities. This initiative has evolved into a very useful twice-a-year publication that is written, read and edited by the local midwives and nurses. It has proved to also be motivating and supporting to novice writers, and gives them direct access to local research. This innovation offers one solution to many of the barriers to publication identified in the literature (Parker et al., 2010).

Another issue, and one that will not go away, is that often there is just *too much* information available on a topic. Health professionals could be in danger of 'drowning' in information overload, especially with the growth of resources on the Internet. However, just because there is a lot of information available, does not mean that people will access it. It is often very difficult even for well-educated professionals to make choices about what information is solid and evidence based, and applicable to their work.

We need to be thinking too about the consumers of healthcare or as they are known in some countries the service user. This important group may be in real danger of making critical health choices based on misinformation if they do not access reliable evidence. Consumers usually do not read nor understand the terminology in scientific journals where more reliable information is available. Friends, family or the Internet are more likely sources of health information, often unreliable at best, and sometimes downright dangerous to the overall health of individuals. Sifting out the 'good and reliable' information from the 'bad and unreliable' information available on the World Wide Web is now a challenge in itself for health professionals who have to respond to service user questions.

Today there is a big emphasis on health literacy, so the health professions need to ensure that information of this kind is user-friendly (Cleary et al., 2007) and based on robust research evidence so consumers can make informed choice.

The problem of non-distribution of findings

In addition to the above, I have found that there are too many filing cabinets or computers around the world containing project outputs that are unfinished or incomplete because their results have not been distributed. Most people who have been involved in a substantial project of any kind know about the hard work or 'blood, sweat and tears' that might have been involved in bringing the project to its conclusion. Project processes, from the original conception to the final report, are often convoluted and complex, especially if funding has had to be found to begin with, research ethics approval achieved, or there have been some issues and setbacks along the way.

Frequently, nurses or other health professionals feel a lack of energy at the end of a project and after writing a comprehensive research report, they may not at that point in time be able to focus on a myriad of useful ways to distribute the findings. I have found graduate students also to be particularly susceptible to this. At the end of a postgraduate Master's or PhD degree it is really a common experience to run out of energy, to feel jaded and stale.

This may have happened to you. You have written and rewritten your work numerous times, and just do not want to look at it again. Remember your thesis work may be the biggest piece of research you might undertake in your life, involving years of work and resulting in comprehensive and innovative results. Unless your thesis supervisors or the educational institution insist on journal publications as part of the research journey, it is quite easy to collect your degree, focus on full time work and then forget about it, leaving the thesis to collect dust on the library shelf; such a waste!

In my experience, nurses often think that the last part of the research cycle is getting the results of their work published in one or two nursing journals, and that's it! Nothing more is done with the findings. So let us turn to the practicalities of disseminating information and outline some possible strategies that may help you with your own work.

Strategies for dissemination of findings

I really want to encourage you to share your work in ways that provide maximum value, so I repeat that you need to think ahead. Think about what you want to share and how you are going to do this; start doing this at the beginning and throughout your project, not just at the end when you have your results available. There is an extensive set of strategies you can use to communicate your findings. However, your decision-making about using any of these strategies needs to involve thinking about whether you should share your work broadly to the health disciplines or to specific groups of people who might benefit from your new-found knowledge or skills. In other words, you need to *target* your audience and *customise* your dissemination processes for that audience, whether it is a local, national or international (see Chapters 2 and 5).

It is important to be guided by your audience, what they access and how they access it, as this will help you decide the best way to communicate with them. Of course, the *nature of the topic* that you want to communicate will help determine your best strategies. Along the way do not forget also that the consumers of healthcare are often forgotten when it comes to dissemination; helping people to care for themselves in health and illness is a vital part of healthcare today and establishing effective methods of communicating your research findings as it relates to key groups can also be considered in your dissemination plans. Consumers are now generally more demanding, requesting health information to help them make choices.

Firstly, you can start looking at the evidence-based literature on distributing knowledge (e.g. Dobbins et al., 2002; Addis, 2002; Haines et al., 2004; Cleary et al., 2007; Oermann et al., 2008; Oermann et al., 2010; Parker et al., 2010), because this will give you more of a background into the issues involved and what you need to think about.

Importantly, you need to focus not just on dissemination, but *how the information could be translated into practice*. Next, my view is that there some important key words that I think go across many of the communication strategies you can use to disseminate findings: *clarity, brevity, usefulness, culturally appropriate, timeliness, relevancy to practice* and *evidence based*. If you consider each of these in relation to what you are going to share, this will help guide you in providing good information. As I mentioned before, it is not useful to provide comprehensive research reports to people who cannot understand or use them. Here are some ideas on dissemination, starting with planning strategies at the outset of a project. Let us think about a clinically-based, quality assurance project involving a team of four colleagues. They could make up a simple plan about their timelines and strategies for dissemination of findings involving consultation with all the relevant stakeholders like the fictitious example shown in Figure 14.1.

You can see, in Figure 14.1, that the quality assurance project research team has dates, clear responsibilities for giving and receiving feedback and a comprehensive set of strategies to release information about the project using: protocols, reports and report drafts, emails, notice board flyers, meetings, the computerised hospital information system, press releases, a publication in a local newsletter, education sessions and a publication in an international journal. The team is also clear about who gets first and second author position on publications. Such a strategy is sure to be a great help to everyone involved to understand the new protocols and implement them into practice.

Disseminating results from a research degree

An important and often delayed activity when undertaking a PhD study is planning for the sharing of results. A relatively simple plan that will help the student keep on track with dissemination is needed, and should be agreed upon early in the research proposal stage by both student and supervisor. In many universities this is undertaken as part of an annual learning agreement between them and often a requirement of their programme of study. A fictitious example is shown in Figure 14.2.

Journal articles and brief research reports

As mentioned in Chapters 2, 5, 8 and 9, when looking for a journal(s) to publish in, decide on the one that your target audience reads regularly. Look around your organisation to find journals being read by staff, ask colleagues or

**Heavenly Care Hospital and JB University:
Emergency Disaster Triage Protocols Improvement Project**

Researchers: Nigel Bloomstead (NB), Project Leader; Katherine Kan (KK); Roger Dawson

(RD); Sue Bambridge (SB)

14/5/2012: Release of draft Disaster Report and Protocols to Ward Managers and

Emergency Team (NB)

30/5/2012: Feedback received and alterations made (KK, RD and SB)

15/6/2012: Project Final Report with Protocols due to Directors (All Team)

30/6/2012: Feedback from Directors and Quality Assurance Team

10–11/7/2012: Release of Protocols to Emergency Team through personal email, notice

boards, hospital information system and staff meetings with all shifts (RD and SB)

12/7/2012: Education team briefed to begin sessions for staff (NB and SB)

Mid-July to end August: Director and team meet with agencies to discuss report:

ambulance, police, fire brigade, SES and local health facilities involved

1/9/2012: Press release to radio, television and local newspaper on disaster report and

changes at hospital (KK and RD)

15/9/2012: Release of publications to County Nurses Association Newsletter and the

Journal of Emergency Disaster Care (KK and NB first authors for one publication each,

RD and SB, second authors on one publication each)

19/9/2013: Evaluation Report due to Director (All team)

Figure 14.1 Example of dissemination strategies for quality assurance project.

check with your institutions' librarians to find out what journals are accessed the most.

In addition to journal articles, remember that clinicians in practice often read short reports, written especially for them in popular industry nursing journals, newsletters from their various nursing associations or from their health institutions. If you have published your findings in a good journal and you want to use other dissemination strategies, be careful that you do not breach copyright by repeating exactly the same information in different articles (see Chapters 5 and 12). It is becoming more common that significant research results are released in a brief article, before a major research publication. This also acts in some way as a record of important first findings/results in

---

The life effects of losing a partner:
An exploratory study of widows in Singapore

September, 2011: Submit systematic literature review to Elderly Care Journal and submit abstract for international conference.

June, 2012: Submit qualitative results to Singapore Caring for Elders Journal.

July-September, 2012: Present findings at an international conference on bereavement.

August-September, 2012: Present findings at workshops at X aged care facility; Singapore Senior Citizens' Club; and Singapore Aged Nurses' Association. Try to gain 5-minute slot at 9LK Community Radio. Write up results for *Ageing & Bereavement* clinical newsletter and press release for daily newspaper.

October, 2012: Submit user-friendly research results to *Singapore Elder's Healthy Life Options Newsletter*. Approach Director of Nursing and Clinical Professor to discuss further possible dissemination strategies to staff.

December 1, 2012: Submit completed thesis.

Figure 14.2 Example of plan for dissemination research results by PhD student.

a particular research field, ensuring that credit is given for that in the research community.

But remember, you can write several different brief articles on your project and its outcomes, and distribute them to different organisations, for publication in industry newsletters, or on websites. The main message being again: 'what is the message you wish to convey and who is your target audience?' (Chapter 5). As an example, take a look at research findings on websites such as the Nursing Times (http://www.nursingtimes.net/), where short user-friendly research findings are regularly displayed.

Clinical articles should be brief and to the point, with key findings and recommendations written in key points format. Put in headings and sub-headings that are questions related to practice (e.g. 'How can I use this dressing?', 'What does this mean for my practice?' or 'How can I use these findings?'). Use brief headings for the article, for example 'Does caesarean section prevent anal incontinence?' or 'Potable water can be used in place of antiseptics for wound cleaning'. Such reports could be as little as 500–800 words.

Put a copy of brief research reports and full journal articles on the *notice boards* in your health facility. If you do not have such a notice board, persuade nurse leaders to make one available for information on improving practice. Make sure all *nurse leaders* get a copy of both your full journal articles and your brief articles. Ask them to distribute these to their staff. Give copies of your article(s) to *key researchers or educators* who are experts in your topic area, within and outside of your country. This will draw their attention to your findings, and they may choose to cite your article in their own articles or disseminate the results to their students, thus helping to spread your messages further.

Targeting consumers

If your findings relate to a particular group of people in the community, for example senior citizens, make sure you target this group by writing to the organisations that they might be connected with, sharing a copy of a specially written article. You could also send this to a government or non-government agency like a health insurance company that sends senior citizens regular newsletters. These days with growing numbers of older people, governments are concerned with their maintaining health and well-being. All people who are older citizens in Australia, for example, receive regular newsletters and can access websites that have articles on topics like the health checks you need, pain management, grandparenting and alternative medicines, to name just a few. For examples of articles you could write for such consumers, take a look at the following website: http://www.yourlifechoices.com.au/. Editors of these newsletters are often looking for articles and if you can get published in these, potentially you have a very large audience. Older people often have the time to read catchy, topical articles.

Other print-based material, DVDs, audio material and videos

Depending on your resources, disseminating your findings on printed material, DVDs and videos might be a relevant way for you to proceed, because they are easily accessible to different population groups but are limited by language and literacy, and often are expensive to produce and distribute (Cleary et al., 2007). Audiotapes might be cheaper and also be very useful for those with poor reading skills or who might be visually impaired (Cleary et al., 2007). If your project has involved making a video, you might want to think about uploading it to YouTube on the Internet to reach a wide audience. Whichever medium you choose, ensure that all relevant permissions have been granted to do this depending on the original source of the material. If it has been a team effort, also ensure that there is a general agreement about publishing that work and in that particular medium. It is always a good point to clarify this at the outset of the research or as an ongoing evaluation of the project, together with peer review of anything you wish to convey publicly prior to doing so.

Podcasting

Another way of sending out project results through audio means is by pod-casting, a modern technology that is fast becoming popular. Think of this as an audio version of an email attachment. People can listen to podcasts in a similar way they listen to radio, either through an iPod or a similar device, or by receiving it as an attachment via the Internet. Audio content, for example, can be downloaded to listen to later when you are walking or relaxing. In this way, very cheaply, project results can be sent out and downloaded by interested people, with you acting as your own 'radio' announcer, recording the programme. Have a look at the following website for more information on podcasting: http://www.podcasting-tools.com/what-is-podcasting.htm.

Blogging

Through the use of blogging you can make comments on various websites about many things to do with disseminating findings. A definition of blogging for those who may still be unfamiliar with the term is found on the Webopedia site (http://www.webopedia.com/TERM/B/blog.html) for all things related to the World Wide Web and the Internet.

(n.) Short for *web log*, a blog is a web page that serves as a publicly accessible personal journal for an individual. Typically updated daily, blogs often reflect the personality of the author.
(v.) To author a web log.
Other forms: Blogger (a person who blogs). [Accessed 6 December 2011]

These blogs include critical comments on research findings on clinical practice, or research events like upcoming conferences or workshops, or describing or critiquing various papers that you have read. These days, blogging on a website can be a highly interactive affair with different individuals commenting on the topic following the conversation of the previous blogger. You can also maintain your own personal blog on your own website on a particular topic.

Press releases

Well-written press releases for both local and national media outlets in radio, newspapers and television can be a potentially good way of communicating important information. More often than not, such releases are emailed these days. You will find that doctors or other researchers, policy makers and government agencies often release these, but seldom nurses.

Activity 1

Have a look at recent press releases on health on the Internet or in newspapers. Writing a good press release about the main points of your project takes a short time. Keep it brief, use simple language understandable to the public, one page is preferable, and once distributed to the right outlets, you will wonder why you have not done it before. Make sure that someone you trust carefully checks your press release, and, of course, if your organisation is mentioned you will need to get prior approval for release to the press.

The timing of press releases is important, and should not occur when there are big news stories that detract from attention to your release. Alternatively, they could be released at the time of a conference or electioneering on health. See the simple example shown in Figure 14.3.

Press Release

Do not release before 21 September 2012

Singapore's Widows Need More Support During Bereavement

A recent study has highlighted the plight of elderly widows in our local community who are lonely and depressed after the loss of their spouse. The study found that they are often depressed for up to 3 years after their husband dies and this has bad effects on their health. The sad fact is that there are not enough community carers or support to help them cope after loss, especially if they have no close family. They lose their appetites, have weight loss and do not sleep well, and often do not join in their usual activities in the community. They sometimes fail to look after their health.

The study, completed by Josephine Ling, a nurse studying at Phoenix University, involved 24 widows aged 65–80. Ms. Ling said that more government attention needs to be placed on counselling services since the number of widows is growing today as women live longer than men. She also calls on non-government organisations and charities to offer better support to these women, and for aged care professionals to develop community visiting programs for recently bereaved widows.

For more information contact Josephine Ling, Phoenix University, Singapore. Mobile Phone: 080-221–345; Email: jling@phoenix-uni.sg

Figure 14.3 Example of a press release.

Of course, in all of this release of information you have to make sure that you become confident in yourself and, for some of you, confident in public speaking or speaking on the radio. It may be that some of you are already on a 'register' of some kind with local radio stations and get called upon to speak if possible on current or newsworthy topics related to your field of interest or research.

Nurses often are not good at self-promotion, but it is important for the profession that many of you learn the politics of promoting information. Take a look at the medical profession and see how they have learnt to be a powerful lobby group over several centuries, by regularly bringing the attention of the public and authorities to their work, especially if it has an impact on the health of the public.

Workshops and other group presentations

Depending on your topic and your target audience, presenting your work to groups is a very important way to communicate your work. However, I have witnessed repeatedly that while nurses are terrific at presenting at conferences or workshops, small and large, they may not write a journal publication on the same topic. Nurses may think this might breach copyright, but often such misunderstandings are unfounded (see Chapters 3 and 9 for some ideas on this issue).

Great nurse leaders give their messages in many forms to many different audiences, and there is nothing stopping you from doing this. Putting your name down for an in-service lecture in your hospital or colleagues in the university is just as important as it is to present at conferences and write publications. One strategy is to write your journal article *first, then* develop your PowerPoint presentation or poster, and your accompanying notes for presentation (see Chapters 3 and 9). By the time you come to presenting at the conference, you will find you needed less presentation notes. You will probably have more confidence to speak directly from the PowerPoint slides, because you know the topic much better after having drafted and re-drafted a journal article. If you are reading this and your research is still relatively recent and unpublished (less than 5 years old), do not hesitate to think about and act on disseminating your results. Use the guidance and advice in this book to help you.

Social media

Communication is being revolutionised today and you can reach a wide audience using social media outlets such as Twitter, Facebook, flickr™ and LinkedIn to get your messages across about your project. These social media outlets are inexpensive and accessible, and increasingly are being used by nursing organisations and journals today.

Evidence-based guidelines for clinical practice

There is no doubt that translating evidence into practice through clinical guidelines is one of the most direct ways that new knowledge can be disseminated. This requires considerable effort, but if you believe that your project has produced evidence that should change the way that health information or care is delivered in your organisation then you clearly need to be thinking about how practice guidelines can be altered to reflect this. This means initially discussing this with whoever are the gatekeepers to clinical protocols in your healthcare facility or your association, presenting your findings and recommendations and if they are amenable and can see the potential for improving patient care, working with them then to developing new guidelines of amending current ones and incorporating the evidence-based changes.

Evidence-based guidelines or protocols continually need updating since knowledge changes so rapidly, but once a successful formula in writing these has been achieved in an organisation, the updating should be a relatively simple process requiring good literature searches. We do not need 'to reinvent the wheel' in this, since many associations, and organisations have protocols in place that may be adapted for use with permission. Many are also published in books and guidelines can be found on the Internet, but may need to be culturally adapted for use in various settings. All readers of this chapter are urged to learn more about the writing of such clinical guidelines and practice sheets for health information since this translation of evidence into a usable form for clinicians is very successful.

Remember I have said that the dissemination of information does not necessarily mean that it will be translated into practice. Read about the organisations that are involved in producing evidence-based guidelines for clinical practice and systematic reviews, for example The Joanna Briggs Institute (http://www.joannabriggs.edu.au/) and The Cochrane Library (http://www.the cochranelibrary.com/view/0/index.html) are probably two of the most well-known ones in nursing.

Conclusion

In summary, disseminating knowledge about the findings from your project is a critical step, requiring strategic thinking. This involves you being knowledgeable about your audience and how you are going to reach them. There are many issues, including some not mentioned, that affect the effective and timely dissemination of findings. Some of these are within our control, and others outside of it, but there is no doubt that dissemination of any aspect of your project work requires effort, especially if new knowledge is going to be translated into practice. Kitson et al. (1996) argued that thinking through the dissemination process, and transforming research into practice is a very demanding process. It requires our intelligence, creativity, clinical judgment, knowledge and skills, organisational knowing and endurance. In other words, it requires a lot of hard work but if we are committed to the task it can be one of the most rewarding experiences, to know that your project has made a difference.

References

Addis, M.E. (2002) Methods for disseminating research products and increasing evidence-based practice; promises, obstacles and future directions. *Clinical Psychology: Science and Practice*, 9(4), 367–378.

Cleary, M., Walter, G. & Luscombe, G. (2007) Spreading the word: disseminating research results to patients and carers. *Acta Neuropsychiatrica*, 19(4), 224–229.

Dobbins, M., Ciliska, D., Cockerill, R., Barnsley, J. & DiCenso, A. (2002) A framework for the dissemination and utilization of research for health-care policy and practice. *The Online Journal of Knowledge Synthesis for Nursing*, 9(1), 149–160.

Gerrish, K., Guillaume, L., Kirshbaum, M., McDonnell, A., Tod, A. & Nolan, M. (2011) Factors influencing the contribution of advanced practice nurses to promoting evidence-based practice among front-line nurses: findings from a cross-sectional survey. *Journal of Advanced Nursing*, 67(5), 1079–1090.

Haines, A., Shyama K. & Borchert, M. (2004) Bridging the implementation gap between knowledge and action for health. *Bulletin of the World Health Organization*, 82(10), 724–732.

Kitson, A.L., Ahmed, L.D., Harvey, G., Seers, K. & Thompson, D.R. (1996) From research to practice; one organisational model for promoting research based practice. *Journal of Advanced Nursing*, 23, 430–440.

Oermann, M.H., Nordstrom, C.K., Wilmes, N.A., Denison, D., Webb, S.A., Featherston, D.E., Bednarz, H., Striz, P., Blair, D.A. & Kowalewski, K. (2008) Dissemination of research in clinical nursing journals. *Journal of Clinical Nursing Journal of Clinical Nursing*, 12(2), 149–156.

Oermann, M.H., Shaw-Kokot, J., Knafl, G. & Dowell, J. (2010) Dissemination of research into clinical nursing literature. *Journal of Clinical Nursing*, 19(23–24), 3435–3442.

Parker, V., Giles, M., Parmenter, G., Paliadelis, P. & Turner, C. (2010) (W)riting across and within: providing a vehicle for sharing local nursing and midwifery projects and innovation. *Nurse Education in Practice*, 10(6), 327–332.

Chapter 15
Other Forms of Writing: Letters, Commentaries and Editorials

David R. Thompson and Chantal F. Ski

Cardiovascular Research Centre, Faculty of Health Sciences, Australian Catholic University, Melbourne, VIC, Australia

Introduction

Many journals, in addition to those papers forming the bulk of their material, carry additional features or columns where authors and readers can correspond about the material in the journal or use the journal to present personal views that will interest the readership. Such features include editorials and correspondence and the latter can take the shape of simple letters to the editor or specific commentaries on papers, usually with a right to reply by the authors of the original paper.

Taking the traditional 'hard copy' journal as an example – where everything that it publishes appears in a hard copy, that is, a paper-based version of the journal, whether or not it first appears online – a major issue is space. Journals usually have too much material submitted to them for publication and unless it is part of the journal structure and policy to print other forms of publication, the priority for space is the original contributions and review papers. Many journals, however, do have an option, at the editor's discretion to include items of news or communications such as short reports that they may not normally publish.

Good practice and ethics of critical commentary

Letters and other similar forms of scientific correspondence are frequently written from a critical perspective and that criticism can be of the journal

Writing for Publication in Nursing and Healthcare: Getting It Right, First Edition.
Edited by Karen Holland and Roger Watson.
© 2012 John Wiley & Sons, Ltd. Published 2012 by John Wiley & Sons, Ltd.

itself or of specific papers that have been published. While there is little policy in this regard – other than procedures for dealing with extreme cases where publication ethics have been violated, or appeals procedures against editorial decisions – there is clearly a place for offering an opportunity to offer a critical viewpoint even if it generates further debate.

The publication of editorials, however, offers very different opportunities for dissemination of critical commentary and, while normally the province of the editor, you will find there are opportunities for guest editorials. These are often for individuals who may be invited to write one, or very often editors receive requests to do so from someone who feels very strongly that an issue, such as attrition rates of students or deplorable care situations where they believe there are solutions to, requires wider promotion and generate public opinion. What advice then can be given to potential authors trying to write for publication in these different ways?

Submission procedures for alternative publishing opportunities

As described previously, most nursing and healthcare journals provide an opportunity for authors to submit letters, commentaries and editorials, though the format will vary between journals. Therefore – as with any planned submission to a journal (Chapter 2) – it is important first to read the journal's information for authors, which is usually provided online on the journal website and sometimes, in an abbreviated form, in hard copies of each issue. Regardless of what you intend to write for publication, it is essential that you target your message to the specific audience you have in mind and submit it to the appropriate journal in the correct format. As with any form of publication, if you wish to impart information, make it clear and simple and try to communicate the message to a general reader. You should also consult a recent issue of the journal for style and content if possible. Authors are usually required to complete an author checklist during the submission process to assist them in meeting the basic requirements of manuscript submission and, as with any other submission, a form ascribing copyright to the journal will have to be completed.

Letters, commentaries and editorials are subject to the same copyright as other published articles and, even if the editor has commissioned a piece from you, the journal is under no obligation to accept and publish it. Letters, commentaries and editorials, even invited ones, are reviewed initially by the journal editor and may undergo a peer-review evaluation.

Some journals have dedicated editors for such correspondence or these may be in the domain of the Editor-in-Chief; either way, these are considered important contributions to the journal. As with other contributions, authors should disclose any conflicts of interest. While this is important in original articles and reviews, it is also important where opinions are being expressed, as these may not be neutral and the reader needs to be aware of any potential commercial or even political implications of such contributions. Authors should not be inhibited from expressing their views if they have conflicts of interest – provided their employer allows this – but readers need to know if the possibility for bias exists. Generally speaking, in western democracies such expression of opinion is not prohibited in any way, as this would be a violation of academic freedom; however, these standards are not universal and this is why these types of publishing activities may still be subjected to review.

Whether the submission process is via the editor or via the usual submission processes of the journal, accepted manuscripts are edited in accordance with the journal's style and returned to the corresponding author for approval and this is usually in the form of a proof. Especially controversial or poorly written pieces may require substantial change prior to being sent to production and proof setting. Authors are responsible for the statements made in their papers, including changes made during editing and production (see Chapter 10).

Letters

Letters commenting on, questioning or criticising other recent articles, including responses from original authors, are increasingly being published. They may be published as rapid responses in some journals and magazines, especially those that are published weekly. Letters often express an opinion but should be relevant, interesting and cogent. It is important to ensure that, although letters may take issue with someone's work, they should be respectful and courteous, avoid inaccurate statements and confrontational or inflammatory language and be limited to the issue in a scholarly manner.

Letters that are seen by professionals and members of the public can influence policy, stimulate debate and even begin to reform healthcare. They have the potential to attract the attention of politicians, lobbyists and opinion leaders, as well as those working in the professions the journal serves. Letters are usually meant to be succinct (150-200 words) and are often limited to five or six references. Many journal editors will send the letter to the lead author of the original paper and invite a response if the author desires. If the author does provide a response this is generally not sent back to the individuals submitting a letter to the editor, although this is not without its exceptions.

One of the first sections often seen and read in a journal is the letters column. Based on their author instructions, many prestigious journals, such as *The New England Journal of Medicine* and the *Journal of the American Medical Association* (*JAMA*), seem to consider the Letters to the Editor column in their journals to be as important as any other article. Although many nursing and healthcare journals do not have a section for letters, a letter to the editor is an excellent place to begin writing for publication. *The Nursing Standard*, a UK journal/weekly magazine publishes letters and opinions. Opinions, clarifications and reflections about articles can be valuable to other readers.

Writing succinct letters is harder than you think; try Activity 1.

Activity 1 Writing a letter

Select a topic to write a letter about. You may have some important issue that you wish to share with others or you may have read something that you wish to disagree with or support strongly. Using the advice in Chapter 2 about getting started and also about losing words, write a letter using as many words as you need to express what you want but try not to go over 500 words. Then cut the letter down to 200 words by deciding precisely what the main points are you want to convey and then lose as many words as possible.

Compare your revised letter with one published in a journal that accepts letters from its readers.

Commentaries

Commentaries may address virtually any important topic in nursing and healthcare and are designed to stimulate debate and offer readers an opportunity to publish their views and opinions of an original article. Commentaries should be well focused, scholarly and clearly presented. They are often of general interest and should be stimulating. A commentary is an extended note that sets forth an expert's opinion on the meaning of a study (Jull, 2007).

By definition, a commentary is a series of remarks or observations that should point out the interesting contribution of the study, that is any new knowledge presented, any discrepancies in the study as compared with available evidence or clinical experience and whether and how the findings of the study can best be integrated into practice (what will this mean to patients, practitioners, educators, managers and policy makers). Commentaries should be well focused, scholarly and clearly presented. Writing a commentary is a good way of engaging clinicians in the research enterprise. The length is usually around 500–1500 words with no more than ten references. An abstract is not usually required for a commentary. Try Activity 2.

Activity 2 Commentaries and responses

The Journal of Clinical Nursing (http://onlinelibrary.wiley.com/journal/ 10.1111/(ISSN)1365-2702; Accessed 1 September 2011) has a well-established system of commentaries and responses. Find a commentary and trace back to the original paper and also try to find any responses by the original authors. After reading the commentaries decide if they were constructive and helpful to the reader of the journal and, had you been the original author, would you have been happy with the commentary on your paper?

Discuss with a colleague and, if confident, approach the editor of the journal with a request or inquiry about writing a commentary of an article.

Editorials

Editorials serve many different functions. As such they can provide a forum for proposing innovative ideas, stimulating debate, raising awareness and challenging the status quo. The best editorials are thought provoking and contentious pieces and in writing one you should be prepared to be controversial and to be prepared for criticism or positive support.

Editorials provide commentary, analysis and question on an important and topical issue, for example they may concern a topic that has been covered by numerous recent publications in the journal you are targeting or in other journals of associated disciplines. You may wish to point out an area of neglect or one in need of future research or you may wish to conceptualise common ground that you have elicited from the recent literature.

Importantly, the topic you decide on and the perspective you take must be evidence based, although the writing of the editorial does not need to be overly referenced. Editorials can also provide commentary and analysis concerning an article in the issue of the journal in which they appear. Editorials can be commissioned by the editor or unsolicited through being submitted to the journal and then invariably peer reviewed. The primary audience is usually a general one, depending on the journal's focus and target audience. The length is usually around 1000–2000 words with no more than ten references if any.

As with all these publications, it is usual to include a title page giving all authors' names, addresses, email addresses, phone and fax numbers, as well as statements of competing or conflicting interests, financial disclosures and copyright/licence to publish. You will be required to sign a covering letter to accompany the article. You will receive an emailed acknowledgement of your submission to the journal. Try Activity 3.

Activity 3   Writing an editorial

Have you ever read the editorial pages of a journal? Have you ever considered writing an editorial? Clearly, if you want to write an editorial then you will have to read a few and look at different examples in different journals. As an exercise, take a range of nursing and medical journals and look, first, to see if they do have editorial pages; if they do then decide what kind of editorials they publish. Do the editorial pages appear to be only written by the editor or members of the editorial board, or does the journal allow guest editorials? If guest editorials are allowed then what kind of editorial are they: are they focused on the contents of the journal or do guest editors have an opportunity to publish on a topic of their choosing?

Consider whether you have something to say about a topic or want to take a position on an issue that has not been considered in the main article section. If yes and you believe you have an excellent idea why not contact the editor and inquire what the policy is on writing an editorial in that journal and what guidelines are there to follow? Also ask if they would be interested in your writing an editorial.

'New generation' commenting facilities

By 'new generation' commenting facilities we refer here to online facilities and these can be 'official' or 'unofficial', referring to whether or not they are under the auspices of a journal or not. While most journal content is published online, whether or not it is ultimately destined for hard copy publishing or not, some only publish correspondence, or a proportion of their correspondence, online. The advantage of online publication is speed of publication and the virtually unlimited space available. If the online correspondence comes under the auspices of the journal and individual pieces are published, as such, with a DOI number (Chapter 2) and referenced as journal content then this latter material will be subject to some or all of the processes outlined previously with regard to good practice and guidelines.

On the other hand, a journal may have its own online environment for commenting on papers in the form of a weblog (more commonly referred to as a 'blog') and this provides space for largely unregulated but not properly published comment on papers with the facility to comment on and augment the blog occasionally.

Some blog material is approved before appearing on the website to ensure that it is legal, decent and honest, but with some blogs the content appears instantly; in either case, the message is to think very carefully before writing anything in a blog; do not be discouraged but remember – as with all social media and publishing in general – you may have to live with some words that have written in haste and later regret.

The importance and influence of such 'blogging' has yet to be evaluated, but closely related to it and with some evidence that it is influential is the influence of social networking sites. Facebook is best known and individuals can set these up for research groups or for themselves and, through more specialist social networking sites, for example academia.edu and LinkedIn, can send links to their papers both to increase their online profile and invite comment.

Of particular importance in this regard is the popular and influential social networking site Twitter, and this has already proved influential with regard to comment on recently released research findings and published papers. In addition, journals use Twitter to advertise their content and, by implication, invite comment, as do many individual researchers. Twitter is especially interesting in this regard as it is almost unique in its facilities. Free to register with and easy to set up, it offers 'tweeters' the opportunity to send out 140 character messages – thereby encouraging brevity – including World Wide Web links to 'followers' – that is people who decide to follow the individual person who are also registered Twitter users.

It is also possible to view individual Twitter pages but not to comment unless you are yourself registered. People following an individual can then 're-tweet' their information to their own followers and, thereby, for some topics a very high profile – much of it simply through duplicated material – becomes created on the Internet. Followers can also comment, through their own 'tweet' on those of others and some fierce arguments arise; direct messages to others on Twitter are possible and, for especially long URLs, online URL shorteners are available to help maximise the information sent out on Twitter. We dwell on this phenomenon here as it is new, already influential and, we predict, will continue to gain influence in the scientific community. It is not possible to say whether this influence is benign or malign at this time.

Activity 4

Search the online pages of journals in your field of practice or interest and determine what, if any, kind of social media communication do they have in relation to publishing material from the journal. Access at least two and compare the differences and similarities between them in relation to what they have to say on certain topics. You may wish to offer an opinion on a topic and are encouraged by other responses to make an attempt. Ensure that your comments do not break confidentiality nor publication ethics.

Submission process and good practice

To ensure your best chance at getting a letter, commentary or editorial published you must endeavour to follow the journal guidelines with absolute precision. Just to recap, and as mentioned in other chapters throughout the book, reviewers and especially editors are not pleased to view a submission that has not conformed to what has been clearly and implicitly stated in the journal's guidelines. Remember always to pay utmost attention to citing and referencing other authors' works as relevant to your work as appropriate. No matter how intellectually sophisticated a paper is, there is always a chance of rejection through mere carelessness and not following any guideline or discussion with an editor themselves.

Some journals such as the *British Medical Journal* (*BMJ*) (http://resources .bmj.com/bmj/authors) and others we have noted in other chapters, have resources for authors that specify what the journal publishes. It provides advice on writing, laying out and submitting articles. This includes detailed advice on:

- where to submit an article;
- how to prepare an article (general requirements);
- what to write;
- what will happen to your article (peer review process);
- editorial policies and practices.

Conclusion

Writing for publication of any kind is a skill worth developing, and being able to write about something you and other colleagues may feel very strongly about is a privilege of a society where 'academic' or 'social' freedom is allowed and encouraged. This is important not only for those writing these types of publications but also may well act as an impetus for future development and activity. Good editorials, for example, can stimulate discussion and debate about recent developments and they can also be published not long or immediately after something has happened or they have read which has stimulated them to the point where they believe it is essential that someone makes their view known. Whatever the reason, it is essential that you maintain a professional standard and adhere to the full meaning of publishing ethics guidance.

A good letter, commentary and editorial all have the power to create a stimulus for change or a change itself. It is essential therefore that it is written well and in the right journal for maximum impact.

References

Jull, A. (2007) How to write a commentary – an editor's perspective. *Evidence-Based Nursing*, 10, 100–103.

Further reading

Ince, D. (2011) Systems failure. *Times Higher Education*, 5 May, 32–37.

Thompson, D.R. & Watson, R. (2010) h-Indices and the performance of professors of nursing in the UK. *Journal of Clinical Nursing*, 19, 2957-2958.

Website

Nurse Author & Editor is a free quarterly publication dedicated to nurse authors, editors and reviewers. It offers advice on writing, editing and reviewing as well as finding publishing opportunities. Available at: http://www.nurseauthor editor.com [Accessed 23 April 2012].

Chapter 16

Where Do We Go from Here? Action Planning for Writing and Publishing

Roger Watson[1] and Karen Holland[2]

[1]Faculty of Health and Social Care, University of Hull, Hull, UK
[2]School of Nursing, Midwifery and Social Work, University of Salford, Salford, UK

Introduction

This chapter is deliberately entitled 'where do *we* go from here?' as opposed to 'where do *you* go from here?' This is to convey that, regardless of our experience and success as writers, each time we sit down to write we are, essentially, starting from the beginning with a particular publication.

We all have the same pressures of time and commitments, which militate against good quality writing time and productivity in terms of what we want to write about or, for many of us, have to write about. Regardless of the importance we place on writing for publication, it always seems to come last in our list of priorities. If this is the situation then what can we all do to continue developing as writers and, most importantly, see our efforts in print? As readers of this book you may already have used some of the advice and guidance given to you by a team of very experienced authors and attained that goal of having an article published. Others may have used the chapter content to help them teach others how to keep developing their skills further and attain a goal such as publication in an international journal that has an impact factor. How then can we ensure that more of you reading this book, who have been undertaking some of the activities and gained additional knowledge, now be successful in writing for publication?

What can we do?

First, this book provides some excellent resources for the budding writer and the experienced writer; keep it, or some similar reference book, close at hand

Writing for Publication in Nursing and Healthcare: Getting It Right, First Edition.
Edited by Karen Holland and Roger Watson.
© 2012 John Wiley & Sons, Ltd. Published 2012 by John Wiley & Sons, Ltd.

to be able to refer to it, for example either for checking that you are keeping to publishing ethics or to access resources that you can use in your teaching or supporting others to develop their writing skills.

Chapter 2 provided some advice on getting started with writing and how to keep going until completion. The most important thing in writing is to overcome the inertia that we all experience; therefore, try to set aside some time each day or as frequently as possible for writing and set yourself some achievable goals. Remember to write first and edit later and also to seek some critical review of your writing.

Although this does repeat what was said in Chapter 2, you now need to consider many of the issues raised in the remainder of the book, the information and guidance that contains more advice specific to different types of publications such as original papers, literature reviews and book chapters. If you are sure you want to write but unsure what to write, then there is a wide range of possibilities and this last chapter will be focused on reminding you what is feasible or not to attain your personal or professional goal.

Activities that will support your writing

Writing does not take place in a vacuum. Writing takes place against a background of curiosity, prolific reading and a desire to share your own ideas or those from a group. You will note the phrase 'prolific reading'. Some of you will be considering 'what do they mean?' by this idea that we have to read a lot to be able to write.

Many first time authors begin their journey to successful publication by sitting down and begin writing their paper. They may have a plan, some material from a project they have been involved in and know they wish to write an article.

They set out to do just that but after two or three pages suddenly realise that they may be able to write very well about the specific topic but, as you will have seen in many of the chapters, there has to be a context or background to those articles that have a better chance of successful publication. This is where those of you who undertake that broader reading around the topic, the possible policies that influence that topic and your work will be able to manage this situation much better than those who have not been reading.

We advise you, therefore, to remain curious and read widely. Do not limit what you read either to refereed journals and textbooks. You should read other types of material such as newspapers, magazines, novels and poetry. You will rarely encounter a good writer who is not widely read and who is not currently reading something that interests them. Of course, there has to be some connections made then to what you wish to write about.

Similarly to writing, there is no shortcut to reading; time has to be set aside but, again similarly to writing, this can be achieved in short periods, especially if it is a theoretical book that will offer a different perspective to developing your ideas on a topic. Those of you who have or are undertaking postgraduate doctoral studies will know this issue very well. We have added some useful reference material in the bibliography that supports some of these general issues we are pointing out in this final chapter.

In terms of reading, in today's technological age you also no longer have to be carrying heavy books with you with the advent of online publishing and the possibility of reading novels and articles on your mobile phone or similar electronic equipment. The ability to download non-fiction textbooks onto these items has revolutionised the need to visit libraries in person, for example. You can now access your own work library at home if you work in a university or are a student without actually visiting the building.

Another rich source of ideas can come from attending a conference, and in addition to listening to the conference presentations you may also be able to meet journal editors who are often invited to facilitate writing for publication workshops at these types of events. The workshops are usually specifically aimed at either novice writers or more experienced writers who may wish to attempt a different mode of publication delivery but, regardless of your stage in writing, any workshops and any opportunity to hear directly from editors is considered valuable. You will also have the opportunity to ask questions and you should not miss this opportunity if there is something that you think an editor can clarify for you about the editorial process we outlined in Chapter 10.

Another opportunity that enhances your own writing and editing skills, as seen in Chapter 11, is to become a journal reviewer. This could also be discussed with an editor you might meet at a conference or study day, especially if the journal is linked to your own area of practice. Different journals have different policies on the kind of experience they expect their reviewers to have but make use of every opportunity to find out if at all possible. Reviewing also helps you to read articles that offer new insights into your area of interest and can often trigger further ideas for writing. It can also stimulate some authors to want to reply to the author of the article because they disagree with what they are saying or may wish to add further knowledge on the same topic. This is discussed is Chapter 15. Whatever form of writing you decide to pursue, it does not have to be a solitary experience.

Collaboration

Writing does not have to be a solitary task and, as mentioned, conferences are an excellent place to meet other people with similar interests, who may agree to write with you because they also wish to share their knowledge and experience on the same topic. However, in today's financial climate within a university or clinical setting, attending conferences is not always possible or feasible. This is where collaboration with colleagues within your own organisation is invaluable, both uni-discipline or cross-discipline, with the latter bringing rewards in the breadth of journals that you can write for and of course an opportunity to increase the number of publications written for different audiences. Some issues for you to consider are as follows:

- If you are collaborating with others please make sure that you all agree on a publication strategy. This would also apply for multi-disciplinary or multi-organisation collaborative research projects.
- The ethical aspects of writing for publication were covered in Chapter 12, so make sure that anyone you approach about collaborating will make a significant contribution; do not offer 'gift authorship' to someone who will make little contribution but whose name will look good next to yours – it does happen.
- Do not ask people to make a significant contribution by way of data analysis or significant revision of your manuscript without proper acknowledgement, which can include co-authorship.
- Always agree on authorship order if more than one paper is being written. Often in a large project, key individuals will take a writing lead on a paper, with various other members adding to the content. The main author, however, is the person who will complete the process and make sure that it is seen as a cohesive whole. Reviewers will often comment on the issue that articles appear to be written by two different people with two different writing styles. It is usually because there has not been one person editing the article prior to submission, although it is appreciated that colleagues contributing together to an article will write differently. The important issue is to have a common agreement on this so that no misunderstanding occurs and as has been known, disputes on primary named authorship.
- Provided you deal with these issues properly, you can learn a great deal working with an experienced author both about the specific issues related to the subject you are addressing but also about aspects of writing and expression. Likewise you will see that experienced writers do not always get it right first time and you must not be afraid, in turn, to make suggestions about their writing; as mentioned in Chapter 2.
- Developing the ability, politely and constructively, to offer comment on the writing of others is an integral part of the process of learning to be a writer.

Look for opportunities to write

As the contents of this book make clear, there are many opportunities to write and ways you can convey your ideas in publications. Therefore, do not eschew invitations to write and do not ignore possibilities for writing other than original papers. Original papers tend to be an essential part of developing a career in nursing education, research, practice and management and will be essential to developing a personal CV. They are considered to be the highest form of achievement in academic writing, especially if they publish your research endeavours with the resulting impact on practice in a given field of nursing, midwifery and health and social care.

Due to your experience and expertise on a subject you may also have been approached by a book publisher either to write a chapter in someone else's book or possibly even edit and write chapters in a book of your own. This can be an exciting way for some new authors to learn about writing and publishing, under the guidance of a more experienced author. Books offer a different medium for some people who actually enjoy 'passing on one's knowledge' about a topic to students at all levels of academic study, or being able to convey to more experienced colleagues something new that they could consider in their clinical work.

Activity 1

It may be useful at this stage of reading this chapter to make some notes about what you think you need to achieve for the future with regard to writing of any kind and identify who may be able to offer you some advice and guidance on the way forward or who you think could help you by being a co-author on a paper. You could also discuss with a more experienced colleague who has already written a book, some ideas you have for a new book prior to contacting a publisher.

The main issue here is that you are making a plan and acting on it. Beware, however, of taking too many responsibilities at once, especially if you already have a large teaching or clinical practice workload. Use the guidance in various chapters in this book to help you manage some of the potential issues that occur.

The opportunities, however, to write original papers is not always available as we plan projects, apply for funding and wait for data to emerge from current projects. Therefore, rather than not do anything, identify how else you can get published in editorials, commentaries articles in professional magazines and also by writing book reviews. Quite simply, the more you write, the better you become at writing. As described in Chapter 15, correspondence in the form of letters and other comments and blogs, are increasingly becoming media for the exchange of ideas.

The difference with these types of media outlets is that pieces for publication have to be completed relatively quickly and the pieces themselves tend to be short. Learning to write quickly and accurately is a very good discipline, one much admired in journalists, and being able to produce short succinct pieces quickly requires and demonstrates a high level of skill as a writer. While these types of output are very unlike original papers, reviews and chapters, the skills you learn in writing quickly and briefly are directly transferable to these other forms of writing. There is no particular style of writing that is more suitable to one particular type of publication; there is only good writing, and good writing uses as few words as possible and 'gets it right' in as few drafts as possible. As emphasised in Chapter 2, there is no shortcut to developing these skills.

You may not be especially busy with your writing career at the start; however, success generates further success in writing and as you progress in your career you will find the opportunities increasing and, sometime, the pressure to write more or differently increasing likewise. This brings us to our next important point, that of organising yourself and your writing.

Organising your life as a writer

If you are serious about writing then you will need to make it part of your life; therefore, you will have to make time for it and be organised in your approach to it. We have noted some books and resources, which will offer guidance on different writing media for you, but as with writing, what you find useful to read is also a personal preference. It is recommended that you look at the books highlighted, some of which offer valuable advice on how to organise time as a writer and manage yourself at the same time (see Epstein et al., 2005; Murray and Moore, 2006; Woods, 2006; Hartley, 2008).

One increasingly popular way of maximising your time and life as a writer is to join in a writing group, some of which can be work based and meet in work time or can be external to work where the pressure may be lessened. For some of you this writing life may be unconnected with your professional life, and if this helps with managing to write better or getting more organised then this can only be to your benefit. Writing groups at work are a form of collaborative writing discussed earlier, but are very useful in helping you to focus time on your writing and having made a commitment to the group, much easier to block out time in your busy working life and your diary.

Activity 2

Find out if there is a writer's group in your workplace. If there is not one then consider setting one up yourself as a means of gaining experience and also meeting other like-minded colleagues with similar interests and a motivation to want to write. Invite someone with some publishing record to come and talk to the group at the onset of your activity in order to share their experiences.

Use the chapters in this book as well to help you with some of the discussion and let us know if it helps you attain your goal of getting some of your writing published. This kind of feedback is invaluable to any writer including the both of us, because at some point we will need to evaluate what our chapter authors and we have achieved and if our combined and individual knowledge and guidance has actually helped the readers of the book. We therefore value any feedback, in exactly the same way that you will have when, having submitted your article for publication, you receive the reviewer feedback. How then do some authors keep track on what they are writing, submitting for publication and receiving feedback?

White boards, organisers and efficient use of your computer

Different writers use different ways of keeping track of their projects and, of course, as a busy academic or clinician, you will not only be required to keep track of writing projects, there will be research grant applications and teaching to keep track of too. However, some specific space should be created for your writing projects and some of the following ideas may help with this:

(1) One popular method that you will see in many academic offices is the use of a white board, which is easily visible in the office and checked regularly. Simply making a list of your projects there by title of the manuscript, which journal it will be or is submitted to and the stage in the process it has reached.

(2) If a manuscript is rejected then simply aim to submit it to an alternative journal, remove the details of the rejecting journal and insert the details of the new journal. *Do not forget, however, to read the new journal's author guidelines before revising it for that journal.*

(3) You can annotate reasonable dates by which you would want to check up with the journal if you have heard nothing by that date, although as we have seen in Chapters 5 and 10, many journals now have a system in place whereby you can track where your article is in the editorial process.

(4) Once you have achieved publication (note that this is a positive statement because we believe that if you follow the guidance expressed by the chapter authors in this book then it is possible to do this), it is a good idea to put a line through the information and put a large tick next to it or write '*published*' next to is in large red letters. This positively reinforces your efforts and also lets other see your success. Of course, at some point it will have to be removed but leave it there long enough to remind you that you have had another publishing success.

(5) White boards are suitable to people who regularly visit their offices but many people do not or they travel a lot and also need to keep track of projects. In this case there are organisers and applications for mobile phones that can also be used and these can also be linked to your diary to provide prompts to action at the various stages of the publishing process.

These are some ways of identifying what you are doing, it is also important to ensure that you also have a system for how you organise and manage to store and save your work.

Managing your writing material and outputs

Using your computer and the various kinds of storage available efficiently is also very important. Some people still work with hard copy (that is with actual paper and pen) and maintain filing cabinets and files of manuscripts and published papers. However, while this is suitable for the person who frequently visits their office, it is not suitable for the busy person who travels regularly and, in itself, even for the person who is regularly in their office, insufficient in the digital age.

With very few exceptions, publishers have moved their methods of working into an online or Internet-based system and that includes submission, reviewing, editing and production. Papers are nearly all published online, therefore, it is possible to submit a paper and have it taken through the whole publishing process to publication and never handle a hard copy of the paper itself. This way of working is also influencing the way we access books and also write them. So the same kind of equipment is also essential to store data from your book writing in much the same way, although not all books are published in an only electronic format at the present time.

In addition, you need to take some simple steps to ensure that you do not lose files and that you know what the latest version of your manuscript is. This can especially be a problem if you are writing with a large team. If you are writing with several people then you can either send the manuscript to each person in turn for their contributions and revisions or send it to one of the team and ask them to pass it on to the next person in turn before it comes back to you.

It is a good idea if each person saves the files with some indication that they did it and when and a simple way to do this is to save the file with the date and the initials of the last person to work on it. For example, when Karen and I were writing this chapter together I started the process and then sent a file to Karen saved as Chapter 16 20.10.11[rw].doc and when she had made her contribution she returned it to me as Chapter 16 30.10.11[rw kh].doc. The final version will have a similar title and date, especially important when we finally send the whole book to the publishers, including all the material that is not written into the chapters. All this work, of course, as well as writing and re-drafting your articles, becomes invisible to the reader of your work, as does all the effort that went into the writing, reading and editing.

It is also crucial to keep backup copies of all your files – again ensuring that you can identify the latest version; some of us experience real worries about this and many colleagues have been known to exhibit some interesting behaviours when saving their work, in multiple places and using various technology such as USB data sticks as well as complicated storing files and additional computer hard drives! Some of you undertaking Doctoral studies may also have experienced similar behaviour when concerned about losing important files.

Whatever system helps you it is essential that you give each version a date so that it avoids confusion and a need to re-write when you delete the incorrect version. Older versions can be stored safely until after publication date because, often, references might be omitted in error and queries from the editorial office will require those that are missing.

Tip 1

Be frequent and regular in saving your files and always know, not only what the latest version of the file is but, as you may have several copies of the file - depending on how many times you back it up - then always make sure that you carry out revisions on the file in the same place: that is on a USB flashdrive or on the desktop of your laptop or personal computer. These may seem like very basic points but it is from bitter experience that we share these with you on the basis of several mishaps arising from computer failure while writing, leaving us without a saved version, or leaving flashdrives in airport lounges - never to be retrieved - and colleagues denying all knowledge of having received our latest revisions by email.

Another chapter (Chapter 10) takes you through the editorial process and describes the job of editors and some insight into whom and what they are. Make sure that you study the editorial process - not just from this book as other resources are available - as this will let you see exactly what you need to do with your writing to maximise the chances that, at each stage of the editorial process, it will proceed to the next.

The main message here could be summarised as: presentation is everything; without good presentation your content, however excellent, will never see the light of day in a reputable publication. Pay attention to detail and try to make the work you submit in manuscript form look as much like a scholarly piece of work as you possibly can.

Conclusion

As we said at the beginning of this chapter, writing for publication does not have to be a 'lone journey'. It also does not have to be an onerous chore. Writing of any kind is a challenge but we know from personal experience of writing for different audiences, via different methods of delivery, that the end result of having your work published is a major outcome and also gives one a sense of achievement.

We hope that through reading the chapters in this book, many of you will find that 'first step' to writing in one of the forms we have discussed as an author team. We also hope that those of you more experienced authors find solutions to challenges of your own and also that there is content that you will be able to use in your own work with developing new authors who wish to publish.

Writing for this book as well as being the editors of it has been both a challenge and an enjoyable journey. We wish you every success in writing and publishing for the future.

References

Epstein, D., Kenway, J. & Boden, R. (2005) *Writing for Publication*. London: Sage Publications.

Hartley, J. (2008) *Academic Writing and Publishing – A Practical Handbook*. Oxford: Routledge.

Murray, R. & Moore, S. (2006) *The Handbook of Academic Writing – A Fresh Approach*. Maidenhead: Open University Press.

Woods, P. (2006) *Successful Writing for Qualitative Researchers*, 2nd edition. Oxford: Routledge.

Bibliography

Clark, R.L. (2010) *The Glamour of Grammar: A Guide to the Magic and Mystery of Practical English*. New York: Little Brown and Co.

Epstein, D., Kenway, J. & Boden, R. (2005) *Writing for Publication*. London: Sage Publications.

Giminez, J. (2011) *Writing for Nursing and Midwifery Students*, 2nd edition. Basingstoke: Palgrave Macmillan.

Hames, I. (2007) *Peer Review and Manuscript Management in Scientific Journals*. Oxford: Blackwell Publishing Ltd.

Hartley, J. (2008) *Academic Writing and Publishing – A Practical Handbook*. Oxford: Routledge.

Lamb, B. (2010) *The Queen's English: and How to Use It*. London: Michael O'Mara Books.

Murray, R. (2009) *Writing for Academic Journals*, 2nd edition. Maidenhead: Open University Press.

Murray, R. & Moore, S. (2006) *The Handbook of Academic Writing – A Fresh Approach*. Maidenhead: Open University Press.

Oermann, M.H. (2010) *Writing for Publication in Nursing*, 2nd edition. Philadelphia, PA: Lippincott.

Woods, P. (2006) *Successful Writing for Qualitative Researchers*, 2nd edition. Oxford: Routledge.

Writing for Publication in Nursing and Healthcare: Getting It Right, First Edition.
Edited by Karen Holland and Roger Watson.
© 2012 John Wiley & Sons, Ltd. Published 2012 by John Wiley & Sons, Ltd.

Index

Writing for Publication in Nursing and Healthcare: Getting It Right, First Edition.
Edited by Karen Holland and Roger Watson.
© 2012 John Wiley & Sons, Ltd. Published 2012 by John Wiley & Sons, Ltd.

CPSIA information can be obtained
at www.ICGtesting.com
Printed in the USA
BVOW07s2031050118
504601BV00001B/4/P

9 780470 657829